HOW TO FIGHT PROSTATE CANCER AND WIN!

4th EDITION

RON GELLATLEY N.D.

1998
Cargel Press International

Copyright © 1998 Ron Gellatley N.D.
All rights reserved.
This book is copyright. Other than for the purposes and subject to the conditions prescribed under the *Copyright Act 1968*, no part of it may in any form or by any means (electronic, mechanical, microcopying, photocopying, recording or otherwise) be reproduced, stored in a retrieval system or transmitted without prior written permission.

ISBN 0 646 35514 7 (1st edition, 1998)
ISBN 0 646 35547 3 (2nd edition, 1998)
ISBN 0 646 35547 3 (3rd edition, 2000)
ISBN 0 646 35547 3 (4th edition, 2000)

Published by
Cargel Press International
P.O. Box 484, Helensvale Qld 4212

All correspondence to
P.O. Box 484, Helensvale Qld 4212, Australia
Email: info@cargelpress.com.au
Website: www.rongellatley.com

Designed, printed and bound in Australia

1 2 3 4 5 02 01 00 99 98

Cover Design by
Rhett Nacson

*This book is dedicated to
my dear wife, Peg,
without whose help I probably
would not have made it.*

Disclaimer

The information and procedures contained in this book are based on the personal experience of the author and are for educational purposes only. It is not a medical textbook, nor is it intended to replace your doctor or other health care provider. The publisher and author are not responsible for any suggestions, preparations, or procedures discussed in this book. All matters regarding your physical health should be supervised by a health care professional.

Foreword

You have in your hands a powerful weapon in your fight against prostate cancer. This book also has invaluable information about enlarged prostate problems and how to get it back to its normal size.

It is a very important book for men who realise they are under threat. They don't have prostate problems right now… but when you consider that something like 80% of all men will get a prostate problem it becomes vital reading.

Did you know that just as many men die from prostate cancer as women die from breast cancer? It is just that men don't get the same publicity or awareness… They should!

Prostate cancer is the greatest cancer killer of men. It is public enemy number one as far as we men are concerned.

What you don't know about your prostate can kill you.

Yes, KILL YOU. And I am not kidding!

The idea to write this book came after I fixed my prostate cancer. The specialist medical opinion was that I had incurable prostate cancer.

I refused to accept this sentence of death. I wanted to pluck the black cap off the judges bewigged head. I wanted the sentence commuted to life. A wonderful long life…

I told myself and a few family members and my best friend that I was going to beat cancer in six months. Never mind this rubbish about me being dead in the not too distant future.

I decided I would do whatever it took.

This book is an account of all the discoveries I made.

The most important discovery for you, if you have prostate cancer or an enlarged prostate, is this…

You have a lot more choices than drugs, chemotherapy, radiation or surgery. It's just a pity neither your doctor or specialist knows about them.

These discoveries changed my life. They saved my life.

It is my dearest wish they will help save yours!

This book is not written like a lecturing text book on the prostate gland. It is a free-wheeling conversation between you and me.

We have something very important binding us together.

We both have a prostate problem threatening our very existence… I have found ways to beat it. I want you to beat it too…

My PSA, the antigen used to measure cancer activity in the prostate, was 126. In six months it came down to 0.08. Remarkable? Only if you don't know about the alternatives to the standard medical responses to prostate cancer and other prostate problems.

How This Book Came to be Written

My boyhood friend is a guy called Chris Robinson. He lives in Melbourne, Australia. We both started school together in England when we were four and a half years old. And we have been friends ever since.

We have shared Life's problems, challenges. We have shared Life's rewards. We are as close as brothers. There is only two weeks between us in age…

When Chris found out I had prostate cancer and the awful prognosis he was devastated. And so was his lovely wife, Marlene. He wanted to come up to our place to give me support. But the last thing I wanted at that time was sympathy. It would have made me even more maudlin with self-pity than I was…

Anyway, at the end of the day, when I phoned Chris with the great news that my PSA was normal, his response was that I should write a book and let other men and their loved ones know there are other options.

Chris told me that few men realised there **were** any other options other than standard medical practice. He believed I had a **duty** to reveal the secrets I had learned in my research into my own survival.

And so the idea for this book was born.

As I said, this is no dull-as-dust text book. It is more like a free-ranging conversation about the problem. Sure, I repeat myself at times, just like you would when talking with someone you like…

The information in this book will shake your built-in opinions, which is a great thing for it to do. Firmly held convictions can be like a steel trap that holds us in a death grip. These opinions are like locks on our minds. Stopping new, and quite possibly Life Saving information getting in. They are like firmly barred windows keeping out the sunshine of revelation to our minds.

There are options. There are other choices we can make.
This book tells you about them.

Bless you…
Ron Gellatley N.D.

Contents

1 The Grim Reaper lays his hand on my shoulder 13

2 Things got worse! 25

3 Cancer is a mind game… And anyone can play! 43

4 Here is the secret of beating your negative voice 59

5 Never mind the drugs… What about YOU! 73

6 Here are some things your doctor doesn't know about! 90

7 On the road to recovery 104

8 God is on the side of the big battalions 120

9 Let us turn the tables on cancer! 139

10 This could be the 'Atomic Bomb' of cancer remedies! 157

11 Two incredible substances your doctor has never heard about! And both of these are powerful anti-cancer agents! 174

12 How a little-known 200-year-old system of medicine can help you beat cancer! 183

13	Healers unknown to your doctor	196
14	Here's how to avoid the devastating effects of prostate surgery… The secrets to not getting a prostate problem… ever!	212
15	How to become the irresistible force against which there are no immovable objects!	224
16	Overcoming impotence… the secrets to male sexual vitality and superpotency	239
17	It's all in the mind… or is it?	252
18	Here are the secret herbs and other helpers!	262

List of nutrients 271

It was a beautiful June day, clear blue skies… not a cloud to be seen. But that beautiful June day turned out to be the worst day of my life!

**HOW TO FIGHT
PROSTATE CANCER
AND WIN!**

1 The Grim Reaper lays his hand on my shoulder

That was the month I was told I had a very aggressive cancer of the prostate. It had invaded and taken over 60% of the healthy tissue.

And the specialist, in his report to my doctor, said the cancer was incurable. Time was not on my side.

I THOUGHT IT WAS JUST A ROUTINE EXAMINATION

I have always enjoyed tremendous good health. I have always been very physical. A keen Rugby player in my youth. Also, a Black Belt Judo Champion for many years until I retired from active competition.

I have always exercised, with weights, stretching, playing golf and generally being active.

My diet has always been low in fat and high in fibre. The perfect picture of health. Everyone told me I looked years younger than my age.

But in June, this all changed.

How I found out I had cancer

My lifelong friend, Chris Robinson, phoned me in May to tell me he had had a prostate examination. Everything was fine. But he had been meaning to have an examination for months and months. And finally, after a lot of 'persuasion' by his lovely wife, Marlene, he saw his doctor. And everything was fine.

This made me think. I had no symptoms to speak of. Although I had noticed that if I drank too much wine I had a problem emptying my bladder.

I made excuses to myself to put off the day when I would see a doctor for an examination. I had never seen a doctor for over 30 years... and that was for a broken hand that happened in a Judo contest!

I wasn't on any doctor's panel. I had no idea how one went about seeing a doctor. I really was a babe in the woods medically.

Fortunately, I knew a good local G.P. who I had met a few times socially and I decided I would give his surgery a ring. I did this and to my amazement I was told that he wasn't accepting any new patients.

I could see I was going to have a difficult time finding a doctor to see me... I then told the doctor's receptionist to tell him that it was me who wanted to see him. Could he fit me in?

Luckily, he said he would accept me as a patient and we made an appointment for me to see him.

I have the tests and everything seems fine...

I think a lot of men don't find the idea of having a prostate examination very appealing. In fact, we find it very non-appealing. The idea of someone sticking his finger up your back passage is not something to welcome.

And I think we men put off this critical examination because we are not comfortable with the idea of having someone put a finger in a very private place. The idea is embarrassing! And a lot of men are inclined to find reasons why it is not really necessary.

Men are the worst offenders in this area. Women are subjected to all sorts of probings, examinations, peering into their most private parts… and they put up with it. They also go and see a doctor as soon as they feel there may be problem.

Not so 'Macho Man'. We tend to tough it out.

And then we become our own worst enemy.

For the sake of a temporary embarrassment we delay seeing a doctor. And all too often it is left too late and it is impossible to help. Had we gone earlier, the cancer could have been cured. At worst, even if not cured, the person's life expectancy would have been considerably enhanced. A lot more years of living would have been possible.

Instead, the man goes to an early grave because he kept putting off what he saw as an embarrassing examination. This seems a very high price to pay to save imaginary modesty.

In the light of my experience, I urge all men over 40 to go for at least an annual check up. It could save your life.

A friend of mine has a large chiropractic clinic… and he has a sign in the waiting room that says in large letters 'Famous Last Words… It Will Go Away!'

It won't and it doesn't. It keeps quietly eating away, chewing up healthy cells, taking over your tissues and silently preparing you for an early grave.

At the end of May I was scheduled to go to a Marketing Convention at Surfers with my business partner and friend, Frank Caruso. So I went to see the doctor a few days before I left for Queensland.

I had the digital examination and it was not anything like as bad as I had imagined it to be. Our imaginations sometimes let us down. We put up pictures in our minds of all the unpleasant aspects and convince ourselves we are fine, when in truth we are not.

At the same time, I had tests for my cholesterol, liver function, had my blood pressure taken, reflexes banged and all those things that doctors do in the privacy of their clinics.

Now listen to this. My blood pressure was that of an eighteen year old. Excellent. My chest was fine. Reflexes? If I drop something I can often catch it before it hits the ground. Lungs in top condition.

The doctor thought I was incredibly fit for my age or even for someone much younger.

And best of all, the physical examination only revealed a slight enlargement of my prostate gland and 'no mass'.

I was in the clear and I went off to my marketing seminar as relaxed and happy as you could imagine.

Everything changed when I got back!

When I got back home there was a message waiting for me. 'Would I phone my doctor as soon as I could'.

Still innocent I phoned him up...

Let me explain something for those of you who have not had a prostate cancer test. The doctor takes a blood sample which is sent to a laboratory for testing. They examine the blood for what are called PSA's. PSA stands for Prostate Specific Antigens and they reveal the presence of cancer.

So your PSA number is an indication of how serious a problem you have. The higher the number, the more serious the condition. And let me tell you, I had a friend whose PSA was 60 and he was declared 'terminal' and he obliged the doctor by making it a self-fulfilling prophecy... by dying.

So when you have a PSA test, you hope like crazy there are no antigens floating about, or if there are, there's not very many!

So I phoned my doctor.

As I said, I was quite naive in this area, and when the doctor told me that my PSA test was cause for concern, it still didn't register that I was in trouble.

He had left a letter for me in his surgery. It was addressed to a Urologist who specialised in cancer of the prostate. I didn't realise that he was a cancer specialist. I didn't realise my life was in grave danger.

When the Urologist saw my PSA his jaw dropped and he just gasped 'Gee!'

The Urologist smiled and asked me to sit down. He was still smiling as he tore open the letter of introduction from my doctor. He pulled out the piece of paper inside and the smile immediately disappeared from his face. His jaw dropped and he gasped 'Gee!'

At that moment it dawned on me that I had a serious problem. My prostate was more than simply 'a cause for concern'.

The Urologist then told me I had a PSA of 126. Terrifyingly high. 126! I couldn't believe it. I mean, how could it be that high? High enough to make the specialist gasp in amazement.

He then explained that I would have to have more tests.

I was to present to his clinic in two weeks time to have a more thorough examination of my condition.

Now you can imagine the next two weeks. I tried to tell myself it was all a mistake. There was nothing really wrong. The tests would put me in the clear. But this small hideous voice kept whispering 'You are in BIG trouble. You could DIE!' I kept trying to shove this thought out of my mind.

I have the tests and it is all bad news

I presented myself at the appointed time. The waiting room was full of all these old men with their wives. Their faces were pictures of misery and suffering. They were all waiting for their turn to find out the bad news. And their faces showed they expected the worst!

Then it was my turn.

The room was empty except for this large white machine humming away to itself. There was a couch. I was instructed to take off my pants and pull down my undershorts. 'Lie on your side.'

Then the specialist gently inserted a cold tube up my back passage. Click. Click. That was fine. Nothing to upset me. No pain. No discomfort.

He explained he had taken some photographs of my prostate.

Now he would take samples of tissue so that the laboratory could do a biopsy. They would examine the tissue, test it, and tell us how much cancer was present and how virulent. Was it a killer or was it harmless?

To take samples they use the same tube they used to take the photographs. With one vital difference. It is now like a gun. It 'fires' a small retractable blade into the prostate and takes out a small slice of it.

I lay there wondering what would happen.

I was not left in doubt for long.

Bang! I felt a sharp jab. Bang! another jab that felt sharper. Bang! and yet another jab. It was getting more uncomfortable each time the blade sliced into my prostate gland.

Bang! Bang! Bang! By this time I had had enough. I asked the specialist if he had enough as I was now finding it very uncomfortable.

He was satisfied with the six and that was that... for now!

NOW I GET THE STARK TRUTH ABOUT MY CONDITION

After getting dressed I went back into his office. He then showed me the photographs he had taken of my prostate gland.

He pointed out to me the dark areas that were the cancer. And there were a lot of them! They seemed to leap out at me. Evil, threatening darkness... I felt my mouth go dry and it was a good job I was sitting down.

I tried to cover how I felt with an air of jollity. When I am tired or nervous I always talk more than I should or is necessary. And this time was no exception. Gabble, gabble… anything not to face what I was seeing before my eyes.

My mind was trying to deny the evidence before it.

I could hear him telling me the awful significance of the photographs. He did a small sketch on a pad on his desk. He drew a circle, this was my prostate gland.

He filled it with dots. The dots were the cancer.

And then he drew dots **outside** the circle and this was really frightening.

He explained that the prostate is a capsule. A small, walnut-sized capsule that sits just below the neck of my bladder. The tube from my bladder goes through the centre of the prostate, which in some respects looks a bit like a small donut.

The reason so many men are getting up so often through the night is because as the prostate enlarges it chokes off this tube from the bladder. And then the stream of urine is reduced to a trickle. The bladder does not empty properly, even though you are stood there for what seems an age.

And not being properly empty it soon fills up and sends a signal that it needs to be emptied. And the prostate can grow so big it chokes off this tube completely and the bladder can't empty.

If this happens and the sufferer is not taken to hospital immediately he can die. Yes, that's a fact. The urine backs up into the kidneys and the body gets poisoned with uric acid. So if you find it very difficult to pass urine, get yourself off to hospital as quickly as you can. You are in trouble.

At hospital they will insert a catheter, which is a narrow tube, up through the penis into the bladder to drain off the urine. They will then probably take steps to enlarge the tube to the bladder as a temporary measure before you go in for an operation.

As you can see, you must not mess about if you even suspect

you have a problem with your prostate. As in all cancers, delay is your biggest enemy.

The doctor explained all this with little diagrams. And I realised whilst I thought I had no symptoms, I had actually had clear warning signs which I had ignored. I had noticed my urine flow had slowed down but I put that down to simply getting a bit older. It has little to do with growing older. If you find you are the last one to leave the urinal after being the first there, you could have a problem. Get off to your doctor and get checked out. Don't try to be a super hero. Heroes get killed.

And, as I said earlier, if I had a few glasses of wine, the flow slowed down dramatically. I had put that down to allergy to the preservatives in the wine… how foolish can you be?

The power we have to deceive ourselves is remarkable. Here am I, a trained Naturopath, a Clinical Nutritionist, a Medical Herbalist, a Homeopath… and denying all the obvious symptoms.

'Me? Symptoms of a prostate problem? Rubbish!'

But they were there all the same and I continued to ignore them.

If it hadn't been for my friend Chris having his examination and being found all clear I wonder when I would have gone?

And when I went I had confirmation of my blindness to the obvious.

'No mass. A slight enlargement.' Great! As I thought. No problem really. How wrong can one be?

So as I said, I went off to my seminar happy as a bird. No problems at all.

But now I was sitting in this bare office with the specialist drawing diagrams on a piece of paper that told me I was in terrible trouble.

He looked at me, his blue eyes piercing, and explained the little dots he had drawn outside the circle representing my prostate gland.

The numerous dots he had drawn represented escaped cancer cells!

I stared at these dots hypnotised by them. 'Escaped cancer cells?'

What was going on? I didn't realise they could escape from the prostate gland.

I knew bowel cancer cells metastased to other organs, usually the liver. But I didn't realise cancer cells could escape from the prostate and lodge somewhere else.

I didn't want to know! I had to force myself to look at the drawing. It now took on a terrible look. If this was the case, what could I do?

I was already thinking terminally. And that is what cancer does to you. It focuses your mind on all the wrong things. While outside, the sun is still shining. You can hear the cars going by. Life goes on. Everything is normal. Except for you. Your life is no longer 'normal'. You are being sentenced to death. You will now spend the rest of your limited time in death row.

All wrong thinking... and in a later chapter I will tell you how I took charge of my thinking on the road to health.

But back to the specialist. He explained that the cancer cells can escape from the prostate gland and usually get into the bones. And it seems this is real bad news. Very bad news!

I would now need to have more tests to find out if the cancer cells had escaped and got into my bones.

But first he would send my prostate tissue samples to the pathologist for examination. Just how bad was the cancer? How far had it got into my prostate? Would it confirm the photographs? How aggressive was it? And if so, could anything be done?

The specialist explained the options. Chemotherapy, radiation, various levels of surgery or drugs. None of it exactly cheery or jolly. In fact, very depressing.

This was my **life** we're talking about. Not the weather. Not some abstract thing. Not a stage show. This was real. This was

ME we were talking about. My prostate. The chance that my bones were infected with the dreaded cancer. It was me who was being discussed as the recipient of chemotherapy, radiation, savage surgery or drugs.

This is true horror. Outside the world seems normal. My car is still parked outside by the kerb. People are walking past wrapped in their own thoughts. Everything is going on as usual. Kids going to school. People out shopping. People at work in their offices, factories or workshops. The trees were beautiful in the new Spring clothes of fresh green.

But life wasn't normal any more.

I had cancer. Cancer of the prostate. And that cancer could now be in my bones. Destroying me as I sat listening to the Urologist gently explaining his damned dots that were damning me to extinction.

'Of course, we don't know for sure. We will have to take more tests to find out if the cancer has spread to your bones.'

More tests... more tests. My whole life now seem to revolve around tests, tests, tests! My mind was completely dominated by the fact I had cancer. All my thoughts were now focused on cancer... CANCER. To say I was depressed was not true. I was terrified.

The future that had seemed so bright. The future that stretched out before me had now contracted . It has shrunk. The sun had gone out. The black clouds swarmed around my head. My brain was full of a damp miasmatic fog. I could not think clearly. I was trying to deny the truth.

Heaven knows I didn't want to die. I began to envy people who had sudden heart attacks that killed them. At least they didn't face the prospect of watching themselves die bit by bit. They had one big sharp pain and it was over.

I was going to die a thousand times. I was going to die in pain. Loaded up with drugs to make existence tolerable. From being a fit person, able to be in charge, to a helpless creature at the mercy of drugs. Totally dependent on others to look after me.

I was appalled at the burden that would be thrown on my dear wife.

For her to watch helplessly as my condition got worse. To watch as I lost weight and became a shadow of myself.

I had seen people die of cancer and it is not pretty!

My father died of lung cancer. It took six months to eat him up. He went from 14 stone of muscle to 6 stone of nothing but skin and bones.

He was in dire pain despite being pumped full of morphine. And finally he died.

And now it was my turn! I broke into a cold sweat at the thought.

I now had to go and tell my darling wife the bad news.

I have never believed it is a good idea to 'shield' one's life partner from the truth. Your partner has a right to know the truth. And so I had to take my wife on one side and try to explain to her the situation.

This is astonishingly difficult to do without becoming emotional.

It is almost impossible to talk about your coming extinction in a matter-of-fact way. I tried to put on a brave face. I tried to minimise the danger.

We decided I should get a second opinion. Who knows. the Urologist could have been wrong. He may have been mistaken. It is amazing how the mind twists and turns in an attempt to deny what is happening.

My wife, Peg, embraced me and whispered 'We'll beat it together, darling as we have done everything together all our lives'.

My wife and I have been together since we were in our teens. We have had a wonderful life. Full of love. We have three tremendous children whom we love to distraction. They are all happily married to terrifc partners who we also love dearly. We have seven tremendous grandchildren who we dote on.

We are a very happy family.

And now all this was going to end for me.

I wouldn't see my eldest granddaughter's 21st birthday. I wouldn't see any of my grandchildren grow up. The future I was working towards with my friend and business partner, Frank, would never happen.

I would no longer get the games of golf in with my dearest friend, Chris Robinson. I wouldn't see him or his charming wife, Marlene, again.

Everything was in ruins.

All because of this damned prostate cancer and the fact it could now be in my bones.

But I carried on as normally as I could. I didn't stop working. When people asked me how I was, I replied as always 'Fantastic!'. I hoped my distress didn't show.

But we still hoped that a second opinion would give me a reprieve. We hoped that a second opinion would get me out of 'death row'.

So we made contacts and a second opinion was arranged with a top Sydney Urologist who also specialised in cancer of the prostate.

Another two weeks of waiting to get in, he is a very busy man and then...

I finally got my appointment to see this top Urologist.

As I got into my car to drive the 130 kilometres or so to

2

Things got worse!

Sydney I wondered what would happen next.

Would I find it was all a terrible mistake. There really was no prostate cancer. My life was not ending prematurely. I would realise all my dreams. All my plans would be realised.

But as I was driving to Sydney my thoughts changed. It was true. I did have terminal cancer. As I drove, the cancer was spreading through my body. None of my dreams would now come true. How long did I have left? Did I have enough time to get my affairs in order? Would I have time to make financial and other arrangements for my darling wife?

The black cloud surrounded me. My mind was dominated by cancer. By thoughts of death. Totally negative. Even though in public I put a brave face on things and smiled mechanically, my mind was elsewhere.

I was finding it hard to come to terms with my condition. My mind rejected the idea that I could have terminal cancer. It refused to believe that my future was now no future. 'Not me! No, not me.' My mind kept saying it as though by saying, it could reverse the inevitable.

How I got to Sydney I don't remember. I must have driven on automatic. I didn't want anyone to come with me. I felt I needed to see this through on my own. Sufficient unto the day for other people to have to share the dread knowledge of my condition.

And as usual in Sydney, I drove around the giant hospital looking for somewhere to park my car. This took my mind off things for a while. Every carpark was full. I didn't realise how many people are in hospital never having been a fan of hospitals. All the pain and suffering going on in that great pile. I should have taken comfort from it. But as they say 'My toothache is more important to me than the other person's amputation'. We humans are very self-centred and our own problems tend to drown out everyone else's. And so it was with me.

I finally parked my car in a one hour spot. Should be long enough, I thought. Except I found I was almost half an hour's walk from where I had to be. I hurried along. I hate being late for anything.

I needn't have worried. When I finally found the right building and after several attempts, finally found the Urologist's office, it was packed. I spoke to his charming receptionist who informed me he was running an hour late. A whole hour! So I went down to the cafeteria to get a drink to pass the time. I read the papers lying there. Well, I looked at them without seeing anything.

Have you ever done that? Sit there reading a book or a magazine and suddenly realising you can't remember a word you have read? At that moment concentration on other things was not my strong point.

So I got in the lift and went back to the office. As I sat there looking at all the other people I got to wondering. Why were they here? How many of them had cancer? What did they do for a living? So on and so on. Eventually, the receptionist called my name and I went into the inner sanctum.

I GET THE TRUTH, THE WHOLE TRUTH AND NOTHING BUT...

The Urologist was a charming man. His office was bright and cheerful, but still clinical. He asked me to take a seat and sat opposite me in his leather armchair.

He asked me to tell him in detail about my problem. And I told him blow by blow what had happened and that my PSA was 126.

'Mmmm' was his only comment. Then, 'Do you have the results of your biopsy with you?' No, the other Urologist would have those.

He picked up the phone and spoke with quiet authority to the Pathology Laboratory who had done the tests. It is strange listening to one side of a two-sided conversation. I could hear things like 'Did you do a six pot? What were the results? Mmmm... That so?'

Finally, he put down the phone and turned to me.

He pulled out a chart with brightly coloured sections on it and pushed it forward to where I could see it.

He pointed to the bright colours and indicated that these were illustrations of cancers. He told me that my cancer was a particularly aggressive one. He also told me that on a scale of 1 to 10 it was at least 7. Not good news at all.

He then asked me to do the usual, take off your pants, drop your drawers, hop on the table. I did all these things and had yet another anal inspection of my prostate. 'Get dressed.' So I did and back to the desk.

The Urologist was a very pleasant man and explained to me that it was possible the cancer had escaped from the prostate capsule and lodged itself in the bones. 'What then?' I asked. His reply was that it would be best to cross that bridge when we came to it.

He also went through the options. Drastic surgery. Chemotherapy. Radiation. He told me the truth.

And this may surprise you. There was little difference in the survival rates between those men having the chemo, the surgery, the radiation and those who had nothing. Most tended to die in their seventies but not from the cancer. They died from heart attacks or other diseases.

But I was not happy with the survival time, which tended to be around five years. I was greedy for a lot longer life than five years... but even five years at that moment would have been a bonus.

But these people didn't have a cancer as aggressive as the one I had! So further tests would be needed.

He told me I would have to go and have what is called 'imaging' done. This means they take images of all your skeletal structure. Your spine, your shoulders, arms, legs, your pelvis. And you have to go to a specialist organisation to have this done.

So off I trotted to the place the specialist told me to go. And when I arrived, more questions, more waiting. I was getting sick of the endless waiting, questions, form-filling, signing this, signing that — I wasn't used to the modern world of medicine at all.

Then the receptionist told me I couldn't be fitted in that day and would have to come back at 9 o'clock the following morning. As I lived over 130 kilometres away, this would mean getting up very early in the morning as it was at least a two and a half hour drive to get there.

Then the receptionist looked at my form, noticed my address and told me they had a branch in the town where I lived. She would phone and try to get me an appointment for the next day. She picked up the phone and dialled while I waited apprehensively. Then she turned and smiled and said 'Tomorrow morning at 11 o'clock. OK?'

That was better. I went off and had lunch with my daughter and her husband who both work in the hospital. I was not the best company.

Suddenly, I remembered my car was parked in a one-hour parking spot and here it was, four hours later. 'That's all I need' I thought. 'A big fine for overstaying my welcome.' I was relieved to find that there was no brown envelope on my windscreen... so thankful for that I got in my car and headed back home.

THE NEWS COULDN'T BE WORSE!

The next day I presented myself at the Medical Centre to have the imaging done. The usual form filling, waiting and then I was called in.

I found myself in a large room with about five large machines sitting there, waiting! A smiling and efficient young man explained to me what I had to do. All very easy. Simply lie on the bench absolutely motionless while the camera, or whatever they call it, slides over the part they are imaging.

Isn't it strange. Whenever someone tells a person to keep absolutely still, certain parts of the anatomy will immediately start to itch. In my case it always seems to be my nose.

I lay there and all I was conscious of was my nose. The end of it started to itch like mad. I wondered how long I could hold on before I ruined everything by scratching my nose. It's funny, but here I was in this awful situation, and at that moment all I was concerned about was not scratching my nose. Thankfully, I heard the technician coming and he moved the machine. I quickly scratched my nose before he moved the 'camera' over the next part of my anatomy.

One of the problems I found with having cancer is that people are always doing things to you. They poke and they probe. You listen, they talk. They bring the big guns of technology to bear. And you just lie there, having things 'done' to you.

You lose control. You are no longer in charge of your own future, your own destiny. You become a puppet. Your strings are being pulled all the time by other people. And there is nothing worse than feeling your life has suddenly gone out of control. It is frightening. You feel so helpless and alone. And no matter how other people express their concern, their love for you, you still feel helplessly adrift.

I believe that in all these cases the system itself works to isolate you. It works to make you feel your fate, your whole future depends on others. It is not intended to work like that. I know lots of doctors and they are all caring people. They are all dedicated to saving lives even though all too often their drugs take lives. So it is not the doctors themselves that make you feel all adrift. It is the system itself.

The form filling. The waiting. Appointments have no meaning. Your appointment could be for 9 o.clock, and yet you are still mindlessly waiting at 10.30. You have lost your individuality. You are a number waiting to be called. The doctor has little choice. It is hard for him or her. They cannot afford to get emotionally involved with the people they see every day. They have to appear aloof. Otherwise they would go crazy with all the harrowing diseases they deal with.

And so you feel you have lost control. You come to depend on the doctor. You feel you NEED him or her. You can easily become a dependant. It is the doctor who now holds your future in his hands. Control has left your hands. And, may I say, this is dangerous.

I believe it is dangerous to give control over your life to someone else, no matter how well qualified that person seems to be. Why? Because this closes off your options. You can only see treatment for your problem through the eyes of your doctor or specialist. And they could be wrong!

And, if they are honest, they would tell you they are wrong at times. But the system requires that we believe they and only they have all the power. Anyone outside the medical establishment is labelled a quack. I have heard of people being told that if they consulted a non-medical practitioner, the 'real' doctor would no longer treat them. And for many people this is a terrifying threat.

And so it is important to remember that you can gain control over your own destiny. Your health is your business. The doctor's business is disease. Remember this.

But I must say, at the time I was having the imaging done I was as helpless as the next person. I was insidiously becoming dependent on the system. I believed they had the power of life and death over me. All my hopes and expectations hung on the results of tests. On medical opinions.

And so I obediently lay there as motionless as I could. I turned when told to. I sat up. I lay down. Until finally I was told it was finished.

Go back again into the waiting room until the doctor could see you to explain the results.

So yet again I sat and waited. My mind was in a turmoil. What would the results show? Had the cancer attacked my bones? Was I safe? Was I in mortal danger? I tried deep breathing to keep my mind off what the results would be. I told myself that worrying wouldn't change anything. But I kept on worrying away just the same. I felt even more alone. Even more isolated. Fearful. Apprehensive. Scared to death.

WHEN THE DOCTOR SAW MY IMAGE HIS ATTITUDE CHANGED!

When I went into the doctor's office he greeted me in a friendly way. We shook hands and he invited me to sit down and view the X-Ray-like negatives on a lighted screen.

It is a very strange feeling to see these images. You find yourself looking at a skeleton. There is the skull sitting on top of the curved spine. And you realise you are looking at yourself... without clothes, without flesh. The bare bones, so to speak. Very strange.

The doctor showed me I had arthritis in my knees and shoulder and growing in my neck. Good heavens, what else?

He then said I would need to have more images taken of my pelvis. So back into the waiting room to wait for an available machine. And then in again.

The technician took images with me kneeling up, leaning forward, leaning back, standing up. Then back to the waiting room.

I was now alarmed. Why did I need all those extra images? What had the doctor seen?

I was not long in doubt.

The doctor called me in and his whole attitude seemed to have changed. It may have been my imagination. I was expecting bad news and I got it.

The doctor showed me the images of my pelvis. And there smack in the middle was a large black mass. So it had got into my bones.

He murmured something like 'These prints are not always conclusive'. But I felt as though he was comforting a doomed man. He was just saying hopeful things to allay my fears.

It didn't work. I knew he was faxing the results to the specialist in Sydney and I had to phone for another appointment.

I went back to my office and told my wife, who was waiting, what had happened. And at this point I lost my cool. I broke down.

It was all too much. I had kept it all in. The grim news. The fear. The terror. The feelings of being out of control.

My dear wife held me in her arms and said bravely 'We will fight it together. We have always fought things together and we have always won and we will win this time'. I nodded my head but I didn't agree with her.

So back to the specialist for his opinion

I phoned the specialist to make an appointment. To my dismay I discovered he had gone on holiday for ten days. I couldn't get to see him for at least two weeks.

Two weeks! Two bloody weeks! My thoughts raced round and round like rats in a trap. Two weeks, meanwhile nothing was being done. The cancer was still growing. Still spewing out deadly cells into my body. It was taking over. It was **killing** me and this bloke was on holiday!

As you can see, all my thoughts were about me. No-one else mattered. They were all right, I was the one with the problem. And my problem was about death. Not life and death. Straight out death!

I didn't realise that prostate cancer is really slow growing. It had started out as one cell ignoring instructions from its DNA. This one cell had invaded the next cell. Its DNA had also gone berserk. Slowly, over what could be a period of years, other cells went bonkers too.

And now they had taken over sixty percent of my prostate. And so ten days or two weeks really made no difference. Anyway, the specialist had booked his holiday months before. And with his workload he needed one.

And so once again I presented myself at his rooms.

Do I have bone cancer?

The dominant question now in my mind was whether the cancer had leapt from my prostate into my bones. If, as the doctor at the imaging centre seemed to think, the large mass in my pelvis was cancer, then I was dead. At least that was how my thinking went.

Since seeing the images and getting the impression that the doctor analysing them was looking at me with what seemed to be sorrow, I had been very depressed.

And this is the problem with cancer. When you have cancer you seem to concentrate on all the wrong outcomes. You see yourself dying. You attend your own funeral a hundred times. In fact, you die a thousand deaths. And each one is devastating. Down go the emotions. Black despair takes over. It is difficult to think straight. You even feel guilty if you laugh or feel jolly.

And that is how I was while waiting to see the Urologist.

Eventually I arrived in Sydney. I went through the same palaver trying to find somewhere to park my car. Finally, I found somewhere and took the lift in the private hospital to the fourth floor. Again, his office was packed. Standing room only for the most ghastly show on earth!

So once again I went down to the ground floor to the cafeteria and bought a cappuccino. I had heard the coffee was bad for people with prostate cancer, but I thought 'What the hell, I am dead anyway, so I might as well enjoy what time I have left'.

As I had time to kill, I sipped on the coffee trying to make it last. I picked up the paper and tried to read it. Different people doing the same things to themselves and other people. Divorce. Murder. Robbery. Did anything ever change?

Certainly my world had changed. From being self-assured I was now very unsure of myself. Where I thought I had a secure future it now seemed as though my future was very limited indeed. It was crazy. Here was I, healthy as anything. Everyone commented on my high energy level. Everyone remarked how well I looked. No-one would believe my age, I looked years younger. And yet… and yet here was I with cancer. Everything in tip top condition except my prostate. A gland the size of a walnut was going to kill me.

It all seemed so unfair. One little gland had the power to outweigh everything else that was as healthy as could be. My cholesterol level was below 4. My blood pressure was 120 over 80. My liver function was fine. Despite all this I believed I had been condemned to death by a gland the size of a bloody walnut. Gross!

So I slowly finished off my coffee and even more slowly

made my way over to the lift. As I went up the four floors I wondered how I would feel in an hour after I had seen the specialist?

So I went back and sat down with the other people. Finally, my name was called out and I went into the office and sat down.

The Urologist had my imaging results in his hands and he looked grave. I feared the worst.

The horror of all this is that everything seems so normal. The sun was shining. I could see cars down below taking their occupants about their everyday business. This is true horror. Everyday scene and here are you in the middle being told you are going to die. At least that is what I thought then.

I saw he had the images of my pelvis in his hand. He was pointing to the black mass with a gold pencil. He was speaking but my mind was not paying attention. I had to ask him to start again.

'I can see this large mass here. I have seen these before on other images' he said. 'However, from my experience, I would say this is arthritis and not cancer.'

I felt weak at the knees. Relief flooded over me like a torrent. 'Not cancer! Oh, thank you, thank you' I murmured to myself. 'I can cope with arthritis.' My mother has bad arthritis and she copes. But my Dad had cancer when he was 52. Cancer of the bowel and he lived for another twenty years. Sadly, he died of lung cancer because he smoked something like 50 cigarettes a day. So cancer ran in our family and so did arthritis.

Tough on me, I got both genes. But good the black mass in my pelvis was arthritis. But the thought came to me. A little dark voice whispered 'What if he is wrong? What if it really IS cancer?'

'Are you sure?' I asked. 'Are you really sure?'

The Urologist smiled and said 'As sure as I can be. I have seen images like this quite a few times, and they were always arthritis. I don't see why yours would be any different'.

So I told the small dark voice to shut up and go away.

AND NOW WE HAD TO DISCUSS THE OPTIONS

The most obvious option was surgery. To cut out the cancer from the prostate and hope it was all taken out. But 60% of the prostate had cancer so that made it very risky. Also, my age was against it. The specialist told me prostatectomies were usually performed on men around 40. In my case there was a very real risk that if he operated, the cancer could be released into my bloodstream with disastrous results.

So an operation was out.

He then discussed chemotherapy and radiation. And said that neither was an option as far as I was concerned. He indicated that the only viable option was drugs.

While all this is going on you feel as though it is someone else who is being discussed. I felt sort of detached. I guess this is a defensive measure. Something like the little boy ducking under the bedclothes so the boogieman wouldn't see him. If I can't see it then it doesn't really exist!

The specialist explained to me that the problem was testosterone. The male hormone. It seems that in the prostate there is a substance called 5 hydroxy testosterone that feeds the cancer.

So the way to stop this happening is to stop the body producing testosterone. The drastic surgery method is to castrate the sufferer. Of course, this is non-reversible. Once it is done you are stuck with it.

From my point of view that is not an option at all.

'No, we do it with drugs' explained the Urologist. 'We inject female hormone into you every month and this reduces your testosterone to acceptable levels. Of course, there are side effects.'

These turned out to be 'a lower sex drive'. It is actually no sex drive at all. And hot flashes. Just like a menopausal woman.

There could also be drug reactions that differ from person to person.

In addition to this it was going to be necessary to shut down the adrenal glands because they too produce a certain amount of testosterone.

But if that is done, my adrenal function is depressed then I will have all sorts of other side effects. Your adrenal glands are the source of adrenaline. The 'get up and go' hormone. The 'fight or flee' hormone that pumps blood into your muscles so you can either run like the wind or fight like a fury. It is this gland that determines your energy level.

There is a clinical condition known as hypoadrenia, which means an underactive adrenal gland. And the symptoms of this are lack of energy, loss of motivation, lack of 'fire'.

My life runs on energy. I need to be fired up for all the things I do. Public speaking. Writing. Motivating people. Feeling on top of things.

What would happen when this drug shut down my adrenals?

Would I become a quiet, unassuming person? Would I lose my spirit? My desire to attack problems, my ability to see problems more as challenges? Would I, in fact, be a different person altogether? Someone even my wife, family and friends didn't know?

Would I lose all my energy and find even the most trivial action too much? No more golf. No more weight training. Even work would be difficult. Was that what I had to look forward to if I took this drug?

I was brought back to earth with the specialist telling me that with the adrenal shutdown drug I would need to have regular liver function tests. This is because it could create dangerous proteins in my liver. If that happened I would need to have more drugs to combat this development.

I was finding this more and more difficult to accept.

Going on female hormone was bad enough, but to have my adrenals shut down with the prospect of major problems with my liver.

The outlook seemed gloomy. I began to wonder if the treatment was going to be worse than the disease!

I had known about the female hormone bit and had discussed it with my dear wife. We have always had a romantic relationship all the years we have been married. Her view was she would rather have me alive with a low or no sex drive, than dead with a potent sex drive.

We could still be loving and affectionate. We could still have a great relationship even if sex was not a part of it. What could I say?

These drugs have to go first to the Health Commission

The specialist wrote out his prescriptions for the drugs. One lot were the female hormone ones. Enough to last six months. The same with the adrenal shutdown drugs. Enough for six months.,

The prescriptions would now be sent to the Health Commission and they in their time would send them to me so I could have them made up.

More waiting. More time to think.

As I drove home I was elated that the black mass in my pelvis was probably arthritis. Much better than a large cancer mass. Much better!

But I got to thinking about the drugs.

All my life I have been against drugs. And here I was about to embark on a course of drugs that would change me. Drugs that would affect my body in undesirable ways.

In our modern society it takes a lot of courage to go against medical opinion. Especially when you find yourself in a real life and death situation. Drugs to stop the production of cancer-causing testosterone seemed right and proper. I would be foolish indeed to let my beliefs get in the way of saving my life. That is how my thought ran then.

Because I was running scared. I was in fear of my life. And in that condition, survival at any price was the dominating instinct. So I was prepared to do almost anything at that time to save my life.

The scripts arrived ten days or so later. I then had to make an appointment with my doctor who would administer the drugs. He would have heard from the specialist and would be looking after me from now on.

So I phoned up and made the appointment to see him.

More unwelcome news...

When I got to see my doctor he had received a letter from the Urologist. He read it out and then gave it to me to read for myself.

One sentence leapt out at me. It grabbed hold of me. The sentence said my cancer was incurable. In the specialist's expert opinion the cancer I had in my prostate gland was incurable. They were going to do their best for me BUT...

My doctor who knew me well, was trying to put as good a face on things as he could. 'It seems we will be seeing a lot of each other from now on' he said. 'Not if I can help it' I thought to myself.

I lay down and he injected the female hormone drug into the flesh to the left of my navel. The other drugs I had to get from the pharmacist and take three tablets a day. Three a day until further notice with regular liver testing.

I decided not to take the adrenal drugs. I didn't take the script to the pharmacist. I thought having the injection was bad enough without insulting my body any more.

The hormonal drug caused me to break out in a horrific rash all over my back and arms. My back looked like it was covered in lizard skin. It looked dreadful. And even worse, it itched like crazy.

I went back to the doctor who at first thought the drug had

made me photosensitive. And that means oversensitive to the sun. And this could mean a grave risk of melanoma. At that time it seemed to me that if cancer wasn't going to get me one way, it was going to get me another.

But then we decided it was a drug reaction.

Let me explain what this particular drug reaction meant to me as a Naturopath. It was quite simply my body trying to get rid of the damned stuff. My body was desperately trying to throw the drug out. It had more sense than I did. It didn't want to have anything to do with it. And so I had this horrendous rash.

The doctor gave me a script for cortisone cream, which I threw in the wastepaper basket. It is my opinion that these creams have very limited value. They give very temporary relief and then the problem comes back worse than ever. Rubbing cream on the rash would eventually drive it back into my body. And that could mean even more problems for me. After all, my body was trying to throw the drug out. So what good would rubbing cream on the rash do?

What it would do would be to prevent the body from doing its job. It would prevent my body from rejecting the drug. So I declined to use the cortisone cream. And decided I could put up with the itching.

I had mild hot flashes now and again. But not enough to worry me. My sex drive disappeared. But my wife and I were more loving with each other than ever. We were thankful to be still together. This drama had made us realise, if we needed reminding, how much we mean to each other.

Everything was more. By that I mean, every caress became incredibly important. It could be the last. The specialist said my cancer was incurable. I was on borrowed time. He had also said the only reason I had any life expectancy was because I was so fit. But I was still on borrowed time.

But the touch of my children, the hugs of my childrens' dear partners became even more precious. To hold my grandchildren and feel their warm bodies against mine, to feel their arms around my neck was a blessing. To talk with my friends took on special meaning.

My best friend, Chris, whom I have known all my life, was very distressed when he heard of my problem. His lovely wife, Marlene, gave me some great advice, which I am passing on to you.

'Build up a large fund of happy memories'.

This is wonderful advice to anyone. You don't have to be terminal for this to be powerful advice. It applies to anyone. It applies to everyone. Build up a bank full of happy memories. Deposit happiness in your account every day.

To make an initial deposit, Chris and Marlene organised a holiday for the four of us at Noosa in Queensland. At the time they believed it would be our last holiday together. They too wanted to make the most of what time I had left.

But by now I was getting fed up. I had gone through the self-pity stage. The 'why me?' The 'woe is me' stage. Now I was getting in the mood for a fight. I have always been a fighter.

I loved Rugby when I was younger. I loved the rough and tumble. I loved to tackle hard. I loved the rucks. I loved combat. I loved the heavy body contact. That was my nature.

I took up Judo when I was about 23. Not long after I got married in fact. I became a Black Belt. I was the Open Black Belt Champion of Zambia. I loved the game and made many life-long friends through it. I remember one of the guys, a higher grade than I was, telling someone he hated drawing me in a competition. 'Because even if I am lucky enough to beat Ron, I am so exhausted at the end of it I'm fit for nothing after.'

That was because I put everything I had into the contest. My entire focus was on beating my opponent.

And now my opponent was prostate cancer.

I began to see this as something like a Judo contest with the highest stakes there are, my life. My opponent was cancer, the referee was the Grim Reaper himself.

And I intended to fight. I was no longer prepared to be a 'victim'.

The time had come to fight. I was now angry with myself for giving in to such negativity. Me, the master of motivation. Me, the very symbol of positive thinking. I had been through the valley of despair and now intended to climb back into the sunshine.

I told myself I would beat the prostate cancer in six months. In six months I would be in remission. That was going to be my Christmas present to myself, to my darling wife and to my dear family and friends.

I decided to show that even experts can be wrong. Incurable? We'll see.

So now I took up the fight in earnest. I began to find out all I could about alternative approaches to cancer in general and prostate cancer in particular. I had helped other people overcome cancer, believe it or not. But I had not applied any of that knowledge to my own condition.

After all, I am a Naturopath, a Clinical Nutritionist, a Homeopath, a Herbalist so if I couldn't help myself, who could?

And with a new spirit, I took up the challenge of prostate cancer. And I determined to beat it in six months.

And in the next chapters I will reveal to you everything I found out and what I did. I want you to win your contest. I want to be your coach. I want to be the guy in your corner. I cannot think of anything I would rather have than a letter from you one day telling me that you too beat cancer. You too are now in remission. You too now have a future to look forward to.

There is no doubt cancer is indeed a mind game. And the

3 Cancer is a mind game... And anyone can play!

problem is everybody who knows about your problem adds to your burden.

Of course, no-one does this on purpose. Their motives are entirely the best. They love you. They are grieving for you. They don't want to lose you. And all their thoughts are on the fact that they think they **are** going to lose you.

Oh, yes. They say all the right things. 'Don't worry.' 'She'll be right' 'I'm sure things will turn out fine' 'Keep your chin up' 'Keep fighting' 'Don't give in' and so on.

However, these sentiments are not expressed with conviction. Because they don't really believe deep down that you will be right. They don't think things will turn out fine. Just the opposite. You have **cancer** don't you? How could things turn out fine. Cancer is a killer. Everyone knows that.

KEEP YOUR CANCER TO YOURSELF AS MUCH AS POSSIBLE

Your first instinct when you get the dread news you have cancer is to rush out and tell everyone. Don't do it!

And here is why you shouldn't go out and tell everyone the grim news. They will all send out the wrong 'vibes' to the universe. They will send out thoughts of death and destruction. Loss and sorrow. Grief and misery. They can't help it. That's just the way we are made.

And they will tell other people.

'Have you heard the terrible news about poor old Ron? Yeah, got cancer of the prostate. Poor devil. Who would have thought it. Well, all we can do is keep hoping…' Then a sad shake of the head.

And entirely the wrong message is going out.

And guess what? They tell even more people about your problem.

So now you have twenty, thirty, forty, goodness knows how many people, all feeling sorry for you. All hoping for the best but expecting the worst.

And this is bad news for you.

Because, whether you realise it or not, you will pick up on this and it will influence your thoughts about yourself. And they will be black thoughts. They will not be thoughts of hope and joy. They will not be thoughts of vibrant health. They will not be thoughts of a long and happy life for you.

All the thoughts are the wrong ones.

So who should you tell?

In my case, I told my darling wife, of course. And I told my much loved children. They have a right to know.

I also told my lifelong friend, Chris and his wife, Marlene. Chris is as close to me as a brother and so I believe he had a right to know. But I didn't tell anyone else.

So I was horrified to find that Chris, in his own sorrow and despair about me, had told his three daughters. His daughters are close too and they sent me messages of cheer. 'We are praying for you.' He also told Marlene's family. So now we have a lot more people talking about it.

Shows how easily the news can spread.

But it is not to your advantage.

I didn't tell my business partner and friend, Frank Caruso, about it until much later. And we are very close to each other.

Take my advice. Keep the knowledge to yourself.

I will tell you how the Universal mind works a little later on.

Don't let your doctor kill you!

It is my belief that a lot of people with cancer die because they are killed by their doctor!

Oh, he or she means well. They don't want you to have what they for some reason call 'false hope'. So they gently tell you the 'facts'. And the facts are you are going to die! You are terminal, mate.

Let me tell you a couple of true stories to illustrate what I mean.

Brian had cancer of the liver. He was only 40 years old. His doctor told him he only had about a year to live. And he told Brian how he would know the end was near.

'The whites of your eyes will go yellow. And then you will know your end is near.'

Can you guess what Brian did every morning when he went into the bathroom? Yes, you're right. He examined the whites of his eyes in the bathroom mirror. He was looking to see if they were turning yellow!

And in just over twelve months they did turn yellow and he did die.

But let's go into this a bit deeper.

When I heard the news I phoned and Brian wouldn't speak to me so I spoke to his wife, Barbara. I told her there were things Brian could do to help himself.

I offered to send him diet sheets. I offered to send up herbs for the liver. I offered to send up Homeopathic medicine for his liver.

And do you know what Brian said?

His very words were 'Ron means well, but it's no use, the doctor has given me twelve months. So there is no use doing anything'.

Yes, that is what he said. And the doctor's statement became a self-fulfilling prophecy. Brian obliged him by dying and made the statement a fact.

But the real truth is that it was only a guess by the doctor. He didn't know for sure how long Brian would live. There are so many factors to take into account. Not just the fact of the cancer.

So Brian did nothing to help himself. He took on board the doctor's words that he only had a year to live. So at the young age of 41 he died and left his wife and four children without a father.

I wonder how long he would have lived had the doctor not expressed an opinion that perhaps would have been better kept to himself.

THE DOCTOR SAYS HE DOESN'T WANT TO GIVE 'FALSE HOPE'

If you had tackled Brian's doctor about it he would probably have told you that he was simply giving Brian the facts. He would not want to give Brian false hope!

Let's have a look at this for a moment.

What is 'false hope?' The same doctor would prescribe chemotherapy, radiotherapy, powerful drugs, surgery, knowing the record of success with these methods is not the best.

The patient puts up with all the miserable side effects, the loss of hair, the nausea, the loss of energy in the belief that the treatment is going to fix the problem. False hope indeed.

So the doctors peddle false hope.

But in my opinion, hope is hope. False hope? What is it? It is only false if the patient dies. It is false if the patient doesn't respond!

But is that 'false' hope?

Statistics reveal that patients who have hope stand a much better chance of survival than those who don't have hope. So shouldn't all health professionals be doing their darnest to give their patients as much hope as possible?

At such a vulnerable time surely the patient should be given positive statements that encourage hope. Surely they should get positive messages from the doctor. Never mind so-called reality. Never mind knowing the 'facts'. The 'facts' may be simply opinions.

So do not take these prophecies on board.

Here is another case history for you to think about.

Albert has prostate cancer. His PSA was 60 and it went up to 69. This despite the fact he was on drugs to drown out his testosterone output.

Now listen to what happened next.

The Urologist who was treating him took him off the medication because it wasn't working. And take note of what he said to Albert and his wife of 40 years.

'Enjoy your next birthday (which was about three months away) because you won't be here to enjoy the next!'

Now what effect do you think this statement had on Albert and his wife?

You are right. It completely shattered them.

All hope was taken away.

Any thoughts of a happy old age together was removed in one blow.

And even worse. Albert took this on board. He believes it.

And he will die in less than a year. He is already behaving like a dying man. He has his friends round to have what are almost 'wakes' with the body still alive. They symphathise. They try to be cheerful. (Very hard when you are with a friend who you 'know' is going to die.)

His wife told me he puts on an act when his friends are there. He tries to be as cheerful as he can. But when he is alone, especially during the lonely watches of the night, he is in despair. And wouldn't you be the same?

Let's have a look at this. Firstly, the Urologist had no right to make such a prognostication. There are lots of factors he doesn't know about. There are lots of treatments he doesn't know about.

Secondly, he surely must know that his patient, in this case, Albert, would believe him. After all, isn't he the 'expert'? Albert would be consumed by the powerful and destructive thought he had only twelve months left to live.

But in my case my PSA was 126. This, according to my Urologist, meant I had incurable prostate cancer. He wrote and told my doctor so.

But I got my PSA down to 0.08 in four months.

So even so-called experts can be wrong.

But sadly, Albert is going to prove his Urologist is right. He too will not take any herbals or Homeopathic medicines. He is now in the condemned cell. On 'death row', waiting for the call.

But I know Albert could get help. I could help him. This book could help him. There are secrets revealed in this book that would probably save his life.

But regretfully, Albert will never read this book. After all, why should he. He **knows** he is going to die. His doctor told him.

And what a terrible waste.

MY DOCTOR TOLD ME I HAD INCURABLE CANCER

When I returned to my doctor, who is a very kind and caring man, he showed me the letter from the Urologist expressing the opinion I had incurable prostate cancer.

My response was immediate.

'Don't point the bone at me!' I said firmly. 'I am going to prove him wrong!'

My doctor smiled. He told me that he fully understood my

concern about doctors pointing the bone at patients. Pointing the bone is an Aboriginal expression for cursing people to death.

He told me he usually tried to give people a talk on being positive.

But he said in my case there was little point as he knew I was one of the most positive people he had ever met.

But he did say 'I guess that we will be seeing a lot of each other now you have cancer'.

And I said to myself 'Not if I have anything to do with it'.

So whatever you do, do not let people tell you the bad news about your lack of a future. Do not believe what the so-called 'experts' say about you. No matter how important that person may seem.

The most important opinion is the one YOU have about YOUR future.

READ DOCTOR DEEPAK CHOPRA'S BOOK *QUANTUM HEALING*

Have you ever heard the expression 'selective perception'?

Let me explain. Let's imagine you have always driven a Holden motor car. You have had one for years.

But then for some reason your next car turns out to be a Ford.

Now what happens is, you suddenly notice all the other Ford cars on the road. Before that, you only really noticed all the Holdens, the General Motors cars. But now you see the Fords.

This is because your perception has changed.

Your mind now selects Fords in the traffic for your attention.

And that is how the mind works.

When you find you have cancer your mind will put selective perception into gear straight away.

And this works one of two ways.

You will either find that all the bad news about cancer leaps out at you. You will pick up on newspaper articles about cancer. You will suddenly notice books about cancer. You will pick up on TV programmes about cancer.

And according to your mind set you will home in either the good news or the bad news.

If you have negative selective perception, you will only believe the bad news. If you have positive selective perception you will believe the good news.

So you must be aware of this trick of your mind.

Make sure you have positive selective perception.

Feed your mind the positive, 'you CAN do it' stuff. Fill your mind with hope. Love yourself. Make your life worthwhile. Put value on yourself. Build yourself up. Don't think the 'tear-down' thoughts that will try to destroy you.

And I put myself into the positive selective perception mode.

And in a bookshop I saw Doctor Deepak Chopra's book *Quantum Healing: Exploring the Frontiers of Mind/Body Medicine*.

And this book had a great influence on my vision of how the mind game of cancer should be played!

When I was in the bookshop this book 'leapt out' at me. Even though nowhere in the title does it mention cancer of any kind. But my subconscious mind knew.

My subconscious mind is into selective perception in a big way. As mine is in positive mode, it guides me to all the good stuff. If it were negative it would attract to me all the bad stuff.

Because that is how it works. For everybody.

And one of my deeply-felt missions in this book is to take you by the hand and guide you into the positive mode.

I sincerely want you to win.

I want you to be in glowing health.

I desperately want you to defeat your cancer.

I want you to return to a happy and fulfilled future.

And I sincerely believe you can.

THE INCREDIBLE POWER OF YOUR MIND!

It is a true saying that what your mind can conceive your body can build. Everything we see around us was once a thought.

I don't want to get into metaphysics, but there are ancient cultures that firmly believe even the flowers, trees, everything was once a thought.

And when you think about it, that's not so crazy. Even flowers these days are the product of thought. Look at all the new varieties of flowers, plants and shrubs that you can see in the garden. All produced from thoughts.

Look at the roads that span the globe. The planes that fly thousands of feet above the earth. Look at the skyscrapers towering above modern cities, and the cities themselves. All the products of thought.

Look at the wonder of computers. We now have computers in almost everything. In our cars, in our planes, trains, washing machines, calculators. There seems little these days that isn't controlled in some way by a computer chip.

And all this started as an idea.

We often find it relatively easy to grasp the wonders of material miracles. But we have problems relating to mental miracles.

And yet your mind is more powerful than any computer.

It has been said we only use something like ten percent of our mental capacity. Think what you could do if you could get a handle on the other ninety percent you are not using.

You would be super genius like the world has never seen!

And that ninety percent is sitting there waiting for you to figure out how to access it. It is neutral. It sits there, waiting.

It is like a powerful motor vehicle sitting in your garage. For some reason you don't know it is there. And even when you find out it is there, you don't have a key to start the engine. So it sits there, waiting. All that power. All that energy. Just sitting there. Waiting to be brought to life.

Well, it is the same with your unconscious mind.

It too is sitting there. All that power waiting for you to harness it.

So how do you get the key to unleash your hidden power?

'Thought Become Things' says Deepak Chopra

In his marvellous book *Quantum Healing*, Deepak Chopra illustrates how a thought becomes a real thing. Every thought translates into a neuro peptide. And neuro peptides are physical things.

THE UNTHINKABLE POWER OF YOUR DNA

In this book, Deepak Chopra talks of the power of the DNA in your cells. DNA contains the blueprint for every cell in your body. And it also brings with it the history of every cell there ever was in your genetic line.

This means it remembers your most distant ancestors. It carries those memories forward into the infinite. And that is a remarkable thought.

And what we are today is the result of an accumulation of thoughts and experiences through our lives. We are the living embodiment of our thoughts. What we are is the result of what we have thought and experienced over the years.

You can't see thoughts... but every time you look in a mirror you are looking at the result of thoughts in action. You ARE your thoughts.

Whilst someone with lung cancer can say his cancer is not the result of a thought... how correct is he? The decision to smoke is his or hers. And the result of that thought, that decision, could be cancer of the lungs.

Somehow the DNA gets changed. It no longer orders the production of healthy cells. No, it now orders the production of cancer cells.

And somehow we have to find out how to change that.

Deepak Chopra believes there is a power in the universe that silently orders events. And I too believe that.

Just think about this for a minute. When you were first conceived you were just a single cell. That cell multiplied a billion times. And those cells all diversified. Some were told to become your bones, some your nose, your skin, your organs and so on.

Now the question is this, how did those new cells 'know' which to become? Why didn't they all just grow into a mass of the same cells? Why didn't they all grow into a gross nose? How did they 'know' what their destiny was?

In *Quantum Healing* Deepak Chopra suggests it is the mind, through the DNA, that decides. Your DNA is a master computer programmer. And it is that DNA that for some reason goes haywire and 'tells' your cells to change.

They grow bigger. They demand more body space. They demand more blood. They invade other cells and their communication with their DNA goes haywire too. Now you have cancer.

And it can be anywhere in your body.

Somehow you have to get the message to your DNA to get back on track. It needs a bit of re-programming.

And the only way to do this is through your unconscious mind.

Let me explain something to you. This is a most remarkable concept. Deepak Chopra suggests that the thought process goes on a bit like this. We think thoughts and between each thought there is a tiny gap. This is a gap of silence. You think, pause, you think, pause, you think, pause. And this is the everyday continuing process in all of our brains.

Thought, pause, thought, pause, thought, pause.

And it is through the **pause** that you get to your unconscious mind.

But how on earth do you get through a gap, a pause, that is only a nano second long? It is so short we think we are continually thinking. We are not even aware there are pauses. So how can we get through those gates, through those pauses?

Deepak Chopra tells about the ancient Indian masters who were able to control their thoughts. It took them years of practice. Of meditation.

And meditation is something Doctor Chopra a recommends we all do. He advocates the single mantra type of mediation. It is known in the West as Transcendental Meditation. In this everyone has a single word they repeat again and again. Everyone has the same word. So you have millions of people silently chanting the same word.

And it is believed one day this will change the world.

But as I read this book, which I recommend you get hold of and read, I wondered how could I get through those gaps.

It was urgent. I had to tell my DNA that I was healthy. I had to tell my DNA I didn't have a prostate that was 60% cancerous. I wanted my DNA to re-programme my cells. I wanted desperately for it to use its power to get things back to order.

This sound crackers, I know. But when you find out you have cancer, you focus on anything that may help.

Why not use affirmations?

A thought suddenly struck me. Why not use affirmations to get to my subconscious mind? If I tell myself often enough that I am healthy surely this will finally get through!

There are people who earn a comfortable living teaching others how to use affirmations to change their lives.

The first person to do this in a formal way was a French Scientist called Emile Coue. He lived in the 1800s and became famous through his use of affirmations to change peoples' lives. His famous affirmation was simply 'Every day in every way, I get better and better'.

Simple and effective. To a degree.

People built on this. Whole books, whole libraries of books, have been written about the power of positive thinking. People still pay hundreds of dollars to listen to the masters of postive thinking.

They come away all fuzzy and with warm feelings. They glow with happiness. But usually, it doesn't last.

It is a bit like drugs. You have to get more and more of it to get the same sort of high.

People pay thousands of dollars to go on one course after another. I wonder how many of these people actually get a meaningful life change?

I know people who have paid out over thirty to forty thousand dollars over time going on courses. They come back all fired up. They have seen the light. They now have the secrets of success in the palms of their hands.

But somehow it so often doesn't seem to materialise. They stay the same old people. And because they don't really change, their lives don't really change either.

They are sincere people looking for enlightenment. They are fine people with the right idea.

For some it is a miracle. Their lives do change. They go on to great success. But you and I know plenty of people who seem to be success seminar junkies. They are always looking for the magic method to change their lives forever.

And they spend their lives and their money searching. But seldom finding.

WHY DON'T AFFIRMATIONS WORK AS THEY SHOULD?

There is no doubt it is far better to have positive, healthy thoughts whether you have cancer or not. It is my view that everyone is a great success. Everybody is using the power of the mind to be successful.

'You must be crazy, Ron' I hear you say. 'Look at the poverty, look at the battlers, look at the misery of the world. How can you say people are successful in the face of all the evidence around you? I mean look at people! How on earth can they be described as successful.'

Well, it all depends on how one defines the word 'success'.

Let me suggest this definition of success: 'Success is getting what you are always thinking about'.

Imagine the power of that thought. Success is getting what you always THINK about. Success is the reward for thinking certain thoughts again and again. It is the manifestation in your life of the thoughts and pictures that dominate your thinking.

Not the things you say. But the real you. The you that believes certain things to be true.

So what most people have are problems. Poverty. Lack. Unhappy relationships. Rebellious kids. Sickness. Gloom. Why? Because they have put those thoughts out to the Universal Mind and the Universal Mind in its wisdom believes that is what you want.

So it makes it come true for you.

Give that some thought. It is a powerful message.

You always get what you think about most. And that is powerful. that is real success.

That is the key to your future.

Have you heard the saying 'What goes round comes round?'

What you put out is what you get back.

Every time. No exceptions. The rule applies to us all.

If you can change your thoughts you can change your world.

Believe me. This a Cosmic Law. Look around you!

All these people short of money. All these unhappy people. All these people hoping the lottery will give them financial independence. All these people on Government handouts. All these people out of work… for ever in too many cases.

Why? Because that's what they believe.

They focus on lack. They focus on poverty. They focus on shortage. They focus on not being able to find a job.

And what is more, everything that happens in their lives confirms their thinking.

And why wouldn't it?

It is their thinking that has brought it all to pass.

As Job said in the Old Testament 'What I have feared has

come upon me'. So it was known over two thousand years ago that thoughts affect what happens to us.

And so I had to find a way to change my thinking.

I had to find a way to focus on health, not on the fact that I had so-called incurable cancer.

And the truth is, when you discover you have cancer, that one terrible thought dominates your thinking. It is hard to function normally.

All your emotions are involved. All those strong feelings.

Now I think affirmations are fine but for one thing…

You have to silence your negative voice.

An affirmation I use is 'Look at me… cancer free' Or 'Cancer free… that's me'. Another one is 'Look at me… Healthee!'

But you have to overcome your negative silent voice.

Let's take an example, OK?

You are poor. You find it hard to make ends meet. You have a desperate need for more money. Your life would change dramatically with more money.

So you try affirmations.

You say things like 'I am wealthy' 'Make a million' 'I am successful' 'I CAN'.

And a little voice whispers… 'Rubbish!'

Because deep down you believe it is rubbish. You are trying but you are not convinced life could change just by saying it will.

So despite your affirmation that you are wealthy, you still buy your Lottery ticket. Because deep down you believe that is the only way you will ever get wealthy.

So you have to change your deep-down beliefs. And far too many of these beliefs are false.

Ask yourself how many of your ideas of wealth or lack of it are really beliefs you have thought about. Come on, really thought about.

Aren't most of them taken in almost with our mother's milk?

Let's look at wealth.

Most people are programmed for lack of money from childhood.

'Money doesn't grow on trees.'

'Do you think I am made of money?'

'There is a world-wide conspiracy to stop you becoming wealthy.'

'Rich people are crooks.'

We are quietly programmed to believe if someone is rich they must have stolen the money. We find it hard to believe they got it honestly.

The popular image of a successful business person is that they got rich by cheating people. Whilst that may be true for a few, it is certainly not true for the majority.

People who get rich understand that wealth comes from giving other people what **they** want. So the person who provides services people want, the person who supplies goods people want, get rich.

In other words they got rich by giving service.

What goes round comes round.

You may have heard the Biblical saying 'Cast Your Bread Upon The Waters And It Will Come Back Tenfold'.

This is simply another way of saying that to become wealthy you must first GIVE.

Most people focus on getting.

But how do you change your focus.

How do you make your affirmations work?

How do you shut that negative voice down that is telling you all the wrong things.

I gave this a lot of thought.

I had to find a way to get through the gap between my thoughts.

It was urgent.

I had incurable cancer.

And according to the medical experts, my time was running out!

4 Here is the secret of beating your negative voice

When you have cancer, the nights are the worst.

In the small dark hours you lie there running your own private hell horror movie show.

Your mind is full of images. None of them good.

You see yourself dying. You grieve. Your guts turn to ice.

And a terrible feeling of helplessness grips you. It floods your whole being.

Your partner lies next to you oblivious of your pain and misery. Which is a good thing. It is bad enough you suffering without involving your partner.

YOU CAN CHANGE THE MOVIE!

Now what is important is to realise that you are the audience, you are also the producer, the main actor. You are also the projectionist. And whether you realise it or not, you own the movie theatre.

So what does that add up to?

What it means is you are in charge.

You have the power to change the film. You have the power to change the plot. You have the power to give your private movie a happy ending.

Believe me, you do have that power.

After all, didn't we agree that you wrote the horror script. Didn't we agree that you were the projectionist. You chose which movie to run.

And you chose the horror movie 'Death From Cancer'.

And so, YOU have the power to change the movie. You do have the power to run a different show. You have the power to write a different script.

You can now write a new script. You can now feature the inspiring movie 'How I Beat Cancer Despite The Experts'.

You can see yourself winning. See yourself happy. See yourself free of cancer. It is your movie. Do what YOU want with it.

How I changed the script of my horror movie

As I write this I re-experience all the despair, the pain and the feelings of hopelessness that overwhelmed me.

But once I made up my mind I had had enough of misery, gloom and hopelessness. Once I made up my mind I was going to fight this cancer. Once I decided I would prove the 'experts' wrong. Once I decided I would give myself six months to beat it.

Things changed.

I woke up to the fact that I **could change the script**.

I woke up to the fact that it was I who was in charge. It was me who was producing and running my nightly horror show. I was a kind of voyeur on my own death. Which is a crazy thing to do.

So I decided that if I had the power to write crappy horror movies, I also had the power to cancel the script. Put my movie house under new management.

A new management that only showed positive, happy ending movies.

STOP BEING A VICTIM, FOR HEAVEN'S SAKE

In the process of closing down the horror movie house and re-opening the happy endings films I discovered something important about myself.

I had been seeing myself as a **victim**.

Things were being done to me.

And they were all nasty things.

I had been poked, prodded, imaged and dosed up. I had been fed one way or another destructive thoughts. They wanted to fill me full of drugs. Maybe even give me radiation, or chemo if their drugs didn't work. There had even been mention of cutting off my testicles.

And told I was incurable!

In other words, I was a victim.

And a victim is not in charge. A victim is just that. A victim!

So I decided to put myself in charge.

And one of the first things I had to do was to sit down and consciously re-write the script of the horror movies I was watching.

Here is what I did.

Firstly, to get messages into your subconscious mind, you must get yourself relaxed.

So the first step is to count yourself down into the alpha state.

The alpha state is a brain wave pattern. It has been described as that stage just before sleep. When you are very relaxed you're more open to suggestion.

So all you do is this.

Tighten every muscle starting with your feet. Tense, then let go.

Now the calves, tense, let go. Now your thighs, tense, let go.

Work your way right up to your head. And pay special attention to your face. You will be surprised how tense your face is!

Now count down from ten to one. Ten, nine, eight… Say to yourself 'I am going deeper and deeper'. Seven, six, five 'Deeper and deeper'. Four, three, two, one 'Completely relaxed now'.

Then what I did (and do every night before I go to sleep) was to see myself in a cleansing room. This is a special place where you can drain all poisons out of your body.

I visualised this large bath and a tube running from me into the bath. I saw my body draining out these dreadful poisons. Bad thoughts came out as red goo. The toxins all came out a sickly green. And the cancer cells came out a mixture of blue and red.

And I flushed them all down the the drain.

I could see my body now empty. Like an empty bottle waiting to be filled.

So next I went next door in my private place.

Now what I am going to say may sound odd, but bear with me.

In my private place I have a helper. His name is Michael.

He is tall, bearded and sunburnt. He wears a coarse brown robe tied in the middle with cord. On his sunbronzed feet he wears strong leaather sandals.

And he has a lovely smile that lights up his whole face. He is not handsome. But he has a strong face, full of character. Which makes him handsome.

And if you think this is odd. It isn't.

I did the Silva programme years ago and I had forgotten I had done it. But in my hour of need I remembered!

Perceptive selection at work again.

And in Silva you count yourself down. In Silva you go into your private place. And in Silva whilst in that state a helper comes to you.

Now you can place whatever significance on that you want.

But the fact is this process works for millions of people all round the world.

And it works for me.

And it can work for you. If you let it!

Anyway, to continue...

Michael connects me to this incredible blue white light that is streaming down. He connects it to my head and floods my whole being with this marvellous light.

And I see this light filling my whole body that I had just emptied in the cleansing room.

And do you know what I see this light as?

Do you know what I **feel**?

This blue/white light is the healing energy of the Universe.

It is the wonderful creative energy of the Cosmic Mind!

And it floods my whole being.

And everything changes.

I get this wonderful euphoric feeling. I feel uplifted. My whole consciousness expands and fills the universe.

I become one with the Cosmic Mind.

And you can do it too. All it takes is practice.

A word about my idea of the Cosmic Mind

I am sure that my vision of Michael, the emptying of the poisons and the filling with the healing power of the Cosmic Mind has gone a long way to help me prove the cancer experts wrong.

It is not my intention to get into a religious debate with my readers.

You have your own conception of God, Universal Mind. These are all highly personal. And that is good.

But whatever your concept is, harness that power to help you win.

This universal presence has the power to help you. Tap into it.

Believe me, you really can tap into this power.

Deepak Chopra in his great book *Quantum Healing* makes the point that some power directs the cells to form bones, blood, tissue, brain and so on. He calls it Mind. Whatever one calls it. There is **something**.

The medical view is that we are like machines.

If something goes wrong, fix that part of the machine.

But we are NOT machines.

We are NOT computers.

We, you, are something special. Very special.

And Doctor Chopra makes a very important point in his book.

And it is this.

That same power that directed our growth from a fertilised egg into a fully fledged human being. That power that causes our wound to heal when we cut ourselves. That power that enables us to digest our food. That power that connects our brains to our bodies.

That power that enables even the trillions of cells in our bodies to 'think'…

That same power CAN HEAL US!

And that is a powerful, wonderful thought.

Take it in. Let it flood your consciousness.

That same power CAN heal you.

But what you have to do is to connect with it.

AND HERE IS THE SECRET OF HOW I CONNECT

Once you start taking charge and DOING something, your life changes.

Let me reinforce this message. You are no longer a victim.

Now you feel you have CONTROL.

There is nothing worse for us than the feeling we are out of control.

The captors of prisoners of war know this.

The prisoners are stripped naked. They are forced to go without sleep.

They are bullied and humiliated. Hope is taken away and then given back... and then taken away again.

Even the strongest people have been known to break down under this sort of torture.

And when you find you have cancer you too feel the same. No future.

But once you get the feeling you do have control, things improve dramatically.

And I want you to get that message firmly into your mind.

No matter what it seems, you CAN do something.

Reading this book is part of your positive selective perception.

My friend and partner, Frank Caruso, says everything happens for a reason.

And you were guided to buy this book.

It arrived in time to help you.

So forward my friend... forward.

How to get through the 'gaps of silence' between thoughts that Deepak Chopra spoke about in *Quantum Healing* became an obsession with me.

I knew if I could find a way to dash thoughts of health through these gaps I would be in the winning seat.

I had to find a way to re-programme my DNA in the cancer cells through my subconscious mind.

Deepak Chopra suggestss Transcendal Meditation. I did this years ago and decided to try again.

I sat myself down and relaxed.

I kept repeating the mantra. A single word.

But then I would fall asleep. Deado.

So I thought it was a good idea to meditate, but I didn't think I was getting through to my subconscious mind.

So what now?

Well, once more positive selective perception came to my rescue.

For a long time I have been in favour of using subliminal tapes.

Now what if I could get an audio tape that gave me guided thoughts and at the same time gave me subliminal messages of health and healing?

I needed a tape where I could hear a voice filling my mind with positive thoughts of health and healing.

But I also wanted the same tape to have subliminal messages in between the audible commands.

Subliminal messages are those you cannot hear but your unconscious mind CAN hear.

So a combination of both would be just what I was looking for.

And I found it!

And I believe it has played a tremendous part in my return to health.

"YOU CAN ALSO HAVE THAT TAPE IN YOUR HAND!"

The tape that did so much for me is now available to you FREE. All you need to do is complete the form in the back of this book and post it to Cargel Press with $8.00 to cover postage and handling.

I am extremely happy to be able to provide you with this tape. Because my dearest wish right now is for you to get well. I pray with all my being for you to get well.

What I found was that if my thoughts strayed off course, my subsconscious mind would bring my conscious thoughts back on course.

It was something like having a gyroscopic compass where the gyroscope brings the ship back on course if it wanders off.

I found myself developing a feeling that I was going to win.

No longer were they just words, a pious hope, it was a fact.

I found I was developing a deep conviction I was going to beat the cancer.

As I said earlier in this book, affirmations are great if you can still the still negative voice that says 'You can't do it'. You need to have a positive conviction"I Can!"

And using this tape did just that... now my affirmations could work without the voice telling me they wouldn't.

My whole mind and body was now full of hope and conviction I would win.

And I dearly want you to change your mind and get the same positive feeling. The inner knowledge that you can win.

THIS IS HOW I USED THE TAPE TO CHANGE MY MIND

I will now tell you how I used the tape to change my mind about myself.

With the best will in the world it is very difficult to change your internal mind about your condition.

You try to be cheerful if only for the sake of your family and friends but deep down the fear lurks casting its dark shadow over your life.

So here is what I did.

Every morning I would relax myself down by counting down from 10 to 1.

Then I would switch on the tape and listen.

I repeat each message. Where it says 'You want health. You deserve health', I would repeat to myself 'I want health. I deserve health'.

I did this with all the messages on the tape.

This way I reinforced the positive messages and also stayed in a relaxed state without falling asleep.

And I did the same thing at night when I came home. Straight into my favourite chair and on with the headphones.

It is a good idea to go to the same place each time you play the tape.

This conditions you to expect to relax.

It is important to make sure no-one disturbs you when you are listening to your tape.

No phone call interruptions. No-one coming in to ask you if you know where the TV guide has gone. No interruptions at all.

Make sure you cannot hear the TV or radio.

Get it through to people you are not playing games here.

It is your LIFE we are talking about.

Make this a twice daily habit.

If you want really powerful results you can get an under-the-pillow microphone. No-one can hear this but you.

You can put the tape on a tape recorder with an automatic reverse mode so it will keep playing all night.

You will fall asleep listening to the positive messages. They will continue all through the night. All the right messages getting through to your subconscious mind.

So it can get through to your DNA and re-programme the maverick cancer cells. Sounds crazy, I know, but believe me my friend, it WORKS.

I have a walkman cassette player, and I play the tape when I am washing my car. I play the tape when I am gardening. I play it as often as I can.

Here is something I thought was important.

One night I was dreaming.

In this dream I was telling someone I had cancer.

And listen to this…

A deep voice that filled the heavens boomed 'You do NOT have cancer… you are RECOVERING from cancer!'

And from that moment I know in my innermost being I was on the way to being cured.

What I did you can do.

What happened to me will happen to you… honest!

Just do it.

There is another great book called *You Can't Afford The Luxury Of A Negative Thought*. Well worth you reading and taking in.

In this book the author says: 'If you have what is thought to be terminal disease concentrate on this thought… If 23,000 people die each year from your disease… think about the 100.000 that DON'T.'

Focus on the positive aspects. Ignore the negative. Become one of those who beat it and you can.

Fill your mind with positive thoughts. Echo Winston Churchill who said in Britain's greatest hour of need 'NEVER, never, NEVER give up!'

What inspiring words. Never give up.

MORE REASONS TO THINK HEALTHY THOUGHTS

Here is an interesting story... just listen to this for a moment.

Some Medical students were examining another student's colon. They had a tube inserted through his anus with a light and a little camera. Like all students they were making light of it all. It was a caper.

They were all making cracks about their colleague on the table and comments about his colon appearing on the TV screen.

You can imagine the scene.

Now something strange happened.

A pretty nurse walked by and looked across at the group and at the naked student on the table.

And he blushed scarlet.

And so did his colon!

The students watching the monitor saw the colon darken as it 'blushed' too.

That is remarkable!

And it illustrates something very important for you.

Your body, your tissues, your cells all reflect how you are feeling.

Your emotions affect your cells.

Pause a moment and think of the incredible importance of this statement. Your emotions affect your cells.

Norman Cousins, a famous American author, found out about this. He had been diagnosed as having a terminal disease. According to all the experts there was nothing more that could be done for him.

He was advised to make the most of what little time he had left on this earth. He was told to get his affairs in order and say his farewells to everybody.

But Norman Cousins didn't believe them.

Norman Cousins decided he would influence his cells. He decided he would have 'happy' cells. He believed it was true that emotions affect your cells.

So here is what he did.

He shut himself up in a room with an enormous pile of funny videos. He had *Laurel and Hardy*, *The Marx Brothers* and *The Three Stooges*. Every funny movie video he could lay his hands on.

And he sat and he laughed and he laughed.

He laughed until his stomach ached.

And guess what?

His cells laughed with him.

And he cured himself... he proved the 'experts' wrong.

He lived for many many healthy, happy years.

And all because he thought only happy thoughts. By watching these funny movies he was filling his whole being with laughter. With positive emotions.

So it is important to remember that your emotions affect your cells.

Bad emotions, anger, jealousy, despair all affect your cells... and in so doing, affect the outcome.

I tell you this to emphasis the need for you to listen to the tape with this book as often as you can.

Make it a habit. It is not something to do 'when you have time'.

Time is precious. You have to make every second work for you.

So listen to your tape at least twice a day. More often if you can.

If you find yourself getting irritable or angry — absolutely the worst emotions for someone with cancer (and for someone who doesn't want to get cancer), here is a little exercise for you.

Smile with your eyes.

Go on, try it. Smile just with your eyes.

It is impossible to feel angry if your eyes are smiling.

Try it for yourself.

Crinkle up your eyes. Make them sparkle with humour.

Whether you realise it or not, when you do this, your face will change. It will become friendly looking. It will relax. It will become more attractive.

Yes, it will.

Look in a mirror. Watch what happens when you smile just with your eyes. You look better. Go on, try it.

And when you are doing it, have a look at your emotions.

You feel happier, the anger will dissipate. It goes away.

Unless you don't want it to. And then you will find it hard to smile with your eyes.

This is a great exercise.

Remember, your emotions affect your cells.

They especially affect your cancer cells. They hate happy positive emotions.

Cancer is a mind game. There is no doubt about it.

There is a strong school of thought that believes most illnesses are the result of wrong thinking sending the wrong emotional messages to the cells.

And remember, you are programming yourself every day.

What you expect is what you are going to get.

What you constantly think about is what you are going to get.

So be aware of your thoughts.

Read this and the previous chapter at least ten times.

Read the words until they become part of you. Part of your thinking and feeling process.

Practise the exercises every day. Two or three times every day without fail. Keep at it. Your life depends on it.

And now you are taking charge of your life.

You are no longer a victim.

Your future is now in your hands. You are doing something positive to put the odds in your favour.

You have had enough of being a victim. You have had enough of hearing how serious your PSA count is. You have had enough of talk of death and destruction.

You have had enough of talks of radiation, radical surgery, chemotherapy, drugs — you are now taking charge of your own life.

Let me tell you, this takes courage.

It will not be easy to overcome the expectations that you will follow the conventional attitude to cancer.

But do me a small favour. Talk to other people with prostate cancer.

What do they radiate? Hope and happiness? Joy and laughter or Resignation?

It is good advice for people who want to be successful in any area of their lives to observe what most people are doing.

And don't do it!

Because most people are not successful.

Most people are victims. Other people and events rule their lives.

I passionately want to help you take charge of your life.

It is YOUR FUTURE we are talking about. Not somebody else's.

So let's get on with more secrets to help you become a winner.

5 Never mind the drugs... What about YOU!

As soon as you are diagnosed as having cancer, whether it is prostate or some other cancer. the reaction is immediate.

What shall we do — drugs, radation, chemotherapy, surgery or do we simply wait and see what happens?

This is a natural and expected response.

Because that is the way doctors are taught. And that is the way doctors think. It is difficult for them to think any other way.

It is interesting to realise that most advances in medicine were bitterly opposed by the mainstream medical fraternity.

When Pasteur suggested that so many women died in childbirth because doctors used unsterilised instruments and didn't wash their hands before they delivered the baby, he was ridiculed.

'Nonsense' 'Ridiculous' 'Absurd' 'Quackery'. These were the cries and they still echo down the years.

When it was suggested that the blood circulated through the body, this too was scoffed at. Poor Harvey, who proposed this theory, was lambasted from pillar to post.

And so it has been down the years with almost every advance.

It is important to realise that your doctor gets no training in nutrition. In fact, it is only very recently that the medical profession would accept that diet had anything to do with disease.

After resisting Pasteur's microbe theory, they then embraced it fervently. They came to believe that germs were the only cause of disease. Kill the germs and you kill the disease.

But unfortunately, it didn't always work that way.

But now the medical profession accepts that in some cases diet could have something to do with disease.

Bear in mind that it has been estimated that six out of ten people in the Western world die from 'diet induced disease'. In other words, poor diet led to breakdowns that then resulted in death dealing disease.

But did you know your doctor has had almost no training at all in nutrition? It is not usually part of the medical training!

And yet, most doctors feel free to pooh pooh vitamins, minerals and other supplements. And this despite the fact they know precious little about any of them.

There are noble exceptions, of course, but the majority of doctors do not know much about nutrition.

And the same applies to Homeopathy, Clinical Nutrition, Herbal Medicine and a whole host of other modalities being used every day to help people.

Now I tell you this not to denigrate doctors. I am not trying to put them down.

No, I am telling you this because you can then understand why your doctor will not tell you what I am going to tell you. And that is because they don't know.

And in many cases, they don't want to know.

It is too difficult for them to believe anything really works outside drug therapy.

Which is a shame.

Do you know, not one of the doctors I have seen about my prostate cancer has asked me how my PSA dropped from a terminal 126 to a safe 0.08 in only five months.

They think it was drugs.

But it wasn't. As I shall now explain to you.

Your body can beat cancer... with help

As a Naturopath the first thing I think of when someone presents with cancer is how to strengthen the host. As an aside, I must tell you that we Naturopaths are not allowed to treat cancer. That is solely the monopoly of the medical profession.

Regardless of results!

So I tell patients I am not allowed to treat them and offer supportive therapy instead. I tell them what I offer is in addition to what their doctor offers. Which is true.

The reason other people are not allowed to officially treat cancer is because the medical profession believes this could delay 'proper' treatment. This in turn would make it more difficult for them to do anything to help the person with the cancer.

However, let us get on with it.

I believe that my first job as a Naturopath is to build up the host. The host is you. You are the host and the cancer is feeding on you!

A horrible thought, but true.

So we have to do everything in our power to strengthen the body. We have to give our body the weapons, as far as we can, to fight the invader.

And the first line of defence, or attack if you like, is diet.

Let's get one thing straight.

We are not talking here about weight loss. We are not talking about your likes and dislikes. Your sugar craving or your alcohol consumption.

No, my friend, we are talking about your LIFE.

We are talking about your SURVIVAL!

So you have to realise that you will have to do whatever it takes to save your life.

This is serious business.

And so back to our diet.

You must be prepared to change your dietary habits. Not for a day, not for a week. But for ever!

I used to say jokingly to my patients 'If all else fails... EAT!'

And eating properly is part of the discipline that leads to a cure at best and extra years of quality life at worst.

Let's have a look at the average daily intake, shall we?

Breakfast is usually cornflakes, toasted white bread, coffee and for some it is only coffee and a cigarette! To make this worse, breakfast is often eaten 'on the run'. It is not a family affair where everyone sits down and has a chat. Relaxing.

No wonder we so often get off to a bad start to our day.

Sometime during the morning we will snatch a cup of coffee or tea and a biscuit or a piece of cake.

Lunch is often a sandwich. And these vary enormously.

Some have salad. Some have different sorts of meat. Some have hamburgers.

The evening meal is usually meat, potatoes and a few vegies. If anything is left on the plate, it will often be the vegies. The meat and potatoes and gravy go but not the vegies.

If you sit down and analyse this daily consumption it is woefully short of vitamins and minerals and trace elements.

The cereals are often loaded with sugars of different kinds. I once examined a packet of 'Natural Muesli' and was amazed at the sugar content.

It had glucose, sucrose, maltose and honey in it. Four different sugars and this was sold as a 'natural' muesli. It may have been the manufacturer's idea of natural, but I can tell you it isn't healthy.

Learn to read labels. The ingredients are supposed to be in order of quantity in the product. Thus the first one is the most and so on down the list.

If you look at cordial, as an example, you will see that water is listed first. So the water is the largest ingredient. Then comes sugar. So next to water you have a heap of sugar. Then comes colouring, preservatives and artifical flavourings.

Definitely not a health drink!

And this is the way all packaged products should be listed.

You cannot afford to take in artificial colourings, preservatives and the like. They are all a burden to your body.

Too much modern food brings nothing with it except calories.

White bread does not have any vitamins in it to digest it. So your body must drag them from somewhere else. And this puts a strain on your body.

And this is the last thing you want.

Your body is fighting for survival. All its energy is needed to overcome the enemy within.

Your body needs foods that build it up.

It doesn't need foods that break it down.

It doesn't need sugar. It doesn't need chemicals. It doesn't need alcohol. It doesn't need tobacco.

These are products that break down your body.

What your body needs are vitamin and mineral rich foods. It needs less meat and potatoes and more vegetables and fruit. It needs nuts, seeds and legumes. It needs foods as close to Nature as you can get.

Do not boil your vegetables. This takes out any vitamins and minerals and washes them down the sink. You need them, not your sink!

Eat them as near raw as you can. Wok them, steam them. But don't boil them.

Reduce your meat and dairy intake. Too much of either of these is not the best thing for you.

Cut down dramatically on cakes, biscuits and chocolates. If you use salt, do not use the white chemically produced stuff from the supermarket. Get the natural salt. It is grey not white.

It hasn't been bleached. There are no chemicals added to make it flow. And it is healthy. This comes as a surprise to most people because we have all been brainwashed to believe salt is bad for us.

Natural salt is not bad for you. Look for Celtic salt. Look for salt from Northern France. Look for the handgathered natural salt.

We are brainwashed to believe we cannot live without milk. But think about this one. Humans are the only species that continues to drink milk after being weaned. And the only species to drink the milk from another animal that bears no resemblance to itself.

For a lot of people milk creates allergies. It can create mucus. People complain of sinus and catarrh, and often they are simply showing the signs of a milk allergy.

Get hold of cookbooks promoting semi-vegetarian diets. Learn to grill your fish, not fry it. Learn to do without greasy foods, so-called snack foods. Read the labels on bottles of drinks from the supermarket refrigerator. You will be amazed at what you find out.

Read them with an additive chart in your hand so you know what the numbers mean.

Your sole aim is to build up your body.

And that is the problem I have with drug medicine. Every drug has side effects. Your body actually tries to resist drugs. The side effects are often your body's reaction in an attempt to get rid of the drugs.

Too many drugs create vitamin deficiencies in your body.

When you are loaded down with drugs, your body now has a two-fold battle.

It has to contend with the disease and it has to contend with the drugs.

Very few doctors focus on building up the patient so his or her body can take part in the curative process.

I realise that some drugs are vital, but all the more reason to build up your body.

So strengthening the host is a major task before us.

CAN VITAMINS HELP, AND IF SO, WHICH ONES?

The 'purists' in nutritional circles believe you can get all your daily vitamin and mineral needs from the food you eat.

They point to the great variety of food available in the modern world. They point out how it is quite possible to get everything you need from your diets.

I do not share this view. And I am not alone. There is a growing number of health professionals who question the attitude of the school of thought that believes we all eat terrific diets.

Let's look at a few examples and see what you think.

Take Vitamin C, probably the best known vitamin. According to the 'experts' you can get all the Vitamin C you need from your diet.

Sure, this could be true if you ate heaps of vegetables and fruit. But most people don't.

It would be true if all fruit and vegetables were full of Vitamin C. But are they? Doctor Michael Colgan did a survey of oranges in America. He took oranges straight from the trees, he took oranges from supermarkets. He took oranges from family grocery stores.

And guess what he discovered?

The Vitamin C content varied from none at all to 375 mg in one orange. And it didn't matter where they came from. So can you really guarantee that if you eat a lot of oranges you will automatically get a lot of Vitamin C?

Have you noticed that when you buy fruit from the supermarket how soon it goes off? That is because so much of it comes from the cold storage depot. It is not freshly picked.

And fruit loses its Vitamin C quite quickly. So does lettuce and other vegetables.

So your chances of building up your body from diet alone is not the best.

You will have to take extra if you are serious about building up your body.

Some more facts about Vitamin C. If you are a smoker, it has been estimated it takes around 30 milligrams of Vitamin C for your body to metabolise one cigarette. So if you are smoking 20 a day you need 600 mg of Vitamin C just to get rid of your tobacco. And how many people who smoke are great eaters of fresh fruit and vegetables?

Remember, the 600 mg is just for the tobacco. You need a lot more for other purposes in your body.

Are you stressed? If you have cancer you are VERY stressed as you know. Under these circumstances your need for Vitamin C goes sky high. You need heaps.

And there is something else to think about. Your cells need Vitamin C as part of their defence equipment. Think of your cells as an army marching to your defence. They have the latest in weaponry to fight the foe. Like an army marching into battle equipped with all the latest technology for destroying the enemy.

And no ammunition!

How do you think they would go on? Not real well!

So when you are stressed, when you are sick, you need lots and lots of Vitamin C. Give your troops the ammo they need!

Now let me tell you something. Normally if you take too much Vitamin C you will get diarrhoea. But it is interesting that when I found out I had prostate cancer I started taking twenty grams of Vitamin C a day. And I didn't get diarrhoea! No matter how much I took I couldn't get to tissue saturation which would have resulted in diarrhoea.

Why not? Because my body is USING it all! That's why!

My body needs heaps of Vitamin C to help it fight the cancer. My body needs heaps of Vitamin C for me to cope with the stress. My body needs heaps of Vitamin C for its anti-oxidant ability.

And I take it by the heaped spoonful two and three times a day.

And I recommend that you do too.

If you are on chemotherapy or radiation therapy, Vitamin C will help your body to cope with the stress. It has been estimated that if you are on these kind of treatments for your cancer you may need as much as 25 grams a day.

I have been told of cases where people who took this amount of Vitamin C did not lose their hair and were not nauseous.

But equally as important is Vitamin C's ability as an anti-oxidant.

Why you need anti-oxidants... every single day

I am sure you realise your body is under attack every day.

Every day your body battles with forces that could overwhelm it. These are called 'Free Radicals'. And billions of them pour into your body every day.

These free radicals have been blamed for almost all degenerative diseases. These include arthritis, ageing, wrinkles and cancer.

Left unattended, free radicals attack your cells. You can see examples of the effect of free radical attacks every day. It is free radical attack that causes iron to rust. Your car bodywork rusts because of free radical attack.

When you start to eat an apple and it goes brown, that is free radical attack too. And this is going on in your body all the time but you can't see it, and you can't feel it. But it is happening just the same.

The windscreen wipers on your car go hard because of free radical attack. And your skin wrinkles and loses its elasticity because of free radical attack.

And it is believed that even diseases like cancer are the result of free radicals attacking the DNA in our cells.

This makes mopping up free radicals a very important part of any therapy to beat cancer.

You need lots of Vitamin C to mop up the free radicals in your tissues.

As I said, I take around twenty grams a day. And I recommend you do the same. If you should get 'the runs', back off a bit. Take ten grams and build up to twenty. Most people find they can take twenty grams without any trouble at all.

So that is the first nutrient in your battle to beat cancer.

You need other anti-oxidants too… believe me!

It is interesting to see that at last the medical profession has accepted the importance of anti-oxidants. In a recent television news item the spokesperson was telling viewers on the air of a man having made a shattering discovery that anti-oxidants really do work.

He was simply telling people the same thing. Naturopaths have been saying for years and years. Previously, we were ridiculed for claiming we need anti-oxidants. Now the medical profession have made them respectable.

Well, my view is better late than never. And with medical approval people who didn't realise the value of anti-oxidants will be more likely to take them. Which could be a life-saver for them!

The major anti-oxidants are Vitamins C, A and E. And the other very powerful anti-oxidant is Grape Seed. I take the original Pycnogenol discovered by Professor Masquelier in France.

I will tell you more about this later, but first let me tell you about the other vitamins, A and E.

Hard evidence proves cancer patients low on A

There is a lot of evidence that indicates cancer patients tend to be low in Vitamin A.

I prefer to get my Vitamin A from Beta-Carotene because I can take a much larger dose. And Beta-Carotene is converted to Vitamin A in your body without any side effects.

BETA-CAROTENE HELPS CANCER PATIENTS

Research has revealed a strong connection between Vitamin A and Carotene intake and various cancers. These cancers range from lung cancer to skin, cervical and others. And even more convincing, research has revealed strong anti-tumour activity in Beta-Carotene.

I read how smokers could help against getting lung cancer by taking large amounts of Beta-Carotene. I was intrigued to read that a large majority of people with cancer had low Vitamin A levels.

And so I decided it would be a good idea to boost my own levels. Which I do. Every day. And I urge you to do the same.

Beta-Carotene has been shown to promote the production of Interferon. Have you heard of this? It is used a lot to combat cancer. But your body itself can produce it given enough Beta-Carotene!

And that is important news for you.

Beta-Carotene helps to boost your immune system and that is vital to survival! Be like me, do everything you can to boost your immune system. It's all to do with strengthening the host (your body) so it can combat the cancer.

Vitamin A has been shown to stimulate numerous immune processes in our bodies. It also stimulates action against tumours. It also boosts the activity of 'killer cells' in our bodies. These 'killer cells' are the ones that attack the cancer. So the more aggressive we can make these, the better.

T cells are killer cells. These search out the enemy in your body and attack. And the Thymus gland produces these killer cells. That is where they get the 'T' from.

But as people grow older it has been found their Thymus gland shrinks. It was thought this was due to age. But evidence now suggests that the real reason is poor nutrition. Vitamin A stimulates the growth of the Thymus gland. Another very important reason to take it.

I see Beta-Carotene, Vitamin A, as an important part of my

attack on the cancer that was killing me. As I keep saying, it is vital that the immune system is boosted by every means possible. And Beta-Carotene is one powerful friend in this fight for life!

As an interesting aside, cancer and aging share a number of characteristics including free radical damage. The good news is that anything that naturally protects you against cancer can also slow down aging. Wow! When I read that I thought 'Well, it ain't all bad news!'

Research has found a relationship between carotenoid content in the tissues and longevity. Here is an interesting tidbit of information.

It has been discovered that humans who reach 90 years have around 50 to 300 mcg/dl whereas rhesus monkeys have a lifespan of 34 years and their carotenoid levels are only 6 to 12 micrograms.

So get into your Beta-Carotene!

VITAMIN E... ANOTHER POWERFUL ANTI-OXIDANT

Vitamin E is a very important vitamin.

It works very effectively to mop up free radicals in fatty tissue.

And as we have agreed, reducing the free radical attack is a major part of overcoming cancer naturally.

Vitamin E gives a kick to cell and body fluid immunity. A Vitamin E deficiency results in a wasting of the lymph system. And an active healthy lymph system is vital to good health.

Vitamin E is also there stopping free radical attack on the Thymus gland. It also boost T Helper cell activity.

What all this means is that we need Vitamin E to stimulate our body's ability to defend itself. And it is never needed more than right now when the body is under life-threatening attack from cancer.

I take at least 3,000 i.u of Vitamin E every single day.

Why? Because I don't want to die from prostate cancer!

A very powerful reason to take daily action to give my body the means to defend me from cancer attack and to prolong my life!

How the humble grape seed is vital to your health

I am a firm believer in a Cosmic Mind. I believe there IS an intelligence out there. Some people call this intelligence by a number of names but whatever it is called, it IS there.

I also believe there are Cosmic Laws. And unfortunately, in spite of our arrogance as human beings, we do not know all of them. We may think we do, but we don't.

And Cosmic Laws are impartial.

They don't take sides.

Break them and no matter who you are, you pay!

It is just like speeding. It is no use telling the traffic cop you didn't realise you were in a speed restricted zone. You were speeding, cop the traffic fine. Ignorance then is no excuse. The policeman isn't interested in your excuses. In fact, if you keep pushing the fact you didn't see the speed sign he will also add 'driving without due care and attention' to your fine for speeding.

And so it is with Cosmic Laws.

Drinking excessive alcohol, smoking, eating fatty foods, eating so-called foods that have little or no nutritional value simply because they taste good. A poor lifestyle breaks Cosmic Laws on health.

Break the Cosmic Law and you pay.

The Cosmic Mind thought of 'play now, pay later' long before the discount houses.

Know that if you break the Cosmic Laws you will eventually get the bill in the form of cancer, athritis, asthma and other degenerative diseases. You may even be called on to pay the unpaid health debts of your ancestors... hereditary disease, they call it.

But what is wonderful is that the Cosmic Mind is forgiving. Change your tack. Straighten up and fly right. Get on course. And you can change your situation.

Trying to cure yourself of cancer while continuing a lifestyle that flouts Cosmic Laws is like trying to empty a bath of water with a hosepipe pouring water in at one end, with the plug out at the other.

And even more wondrous is that the Cosmic Mind has provided us with herbs that can help us. And here we are, destroying them as fast as we can go.

Who knows what treasures are being destroyed every day in the rain forests? And as I said, the Cosmic Mind is impartial.

It provides these wonder herbs. We, in our ignorance, destroy them willy nilly. Tough! We pay!

And locked into the humble grape seed is a dynamite power of anti-oxidant activity.

It contains large amounts of what are called 'flavonoids' and you will be hearing more and more about these as time goes on. A lot of research is going into these substances.

In France, Professor Masquelier has done tremendous research into flavonoids and their effect on human health. He discovered that a rich source was in the bark of the Maritime Pine Tree.

Only one problem. Taking the bark off a tree kills it.

So another source had to be found. And Professor Masquelier found it in Grape Seeds.

He called his discovery 'Pycnogenol'. This was the first of its kind in the marketplace. I first heard of it in America and used to import it for my own use until for some reason export to Australia was stopped.

This was long before I developed prostate cancer. So I was glad to re-discover Pycnogenol here in Australia. And now I take it every day.

These flavonoids are probably the most potent anti-oxidants

in the world today. More powerful than Vitamin C or Vitamin E. You still need Vitamins A and C for other reasons. Although, I must say in my view, the more 'troops' I can throw into the battle the better.

So I take large amounts of Vitamin C, Beta-Carotene, Vitamin E and Pycnogenol.

You can get flavonoids now in many brands. They are sold as Grape Seed in various strengths. I urge you to consider taking flavonoids. I believe they are essential in the battle to boost the immune system. And the immune system is essential in the war against cancer. Boosting the immune system became almost an obsession with me.

I read everything I could lay my hands on. I asked lots of questions. I read and re-read all the various monograms I had received on various aspects of the immune system.

BOWEL FLORA AND THE IMMUNE SYSTEM

Did you know that the bacteria in your bowel are an important part of your immune system? We normally think of the bowel as a garbage disposal system. But as part of the immune system?

Well, there are all kinds of bacteria in your bowel. Good and bad.

The majority of people have too many bacteria of the wrong kind. This happens because of poor digestion. The wrong foods. One problem we humans have is we continue to eat like teenagers when we have the digestion of senior citizens.

And this results in a proliferation of the wrong kind of bacteria.

Want proof? OK. Haven't you noticed how many people as they get older develop wind. They also suffer a lot from indigestion and heartburn.

Pharmacists sell antacid powders by the ton. These are a staple product with the pharmacists. Like potatoes to a greengrocer. People all over the world are crunching tablets, sucking lozenges, drinking white powder drinks. All with the same objective.

To try to calm a stomach that has gone wild. And they never seem to fix the problem. It never goes away. Eating that was once a pleasure now is followed by misery.

Wind so bad it seems like a heart attack. Reflux so bad the person can't lie down in bed. Heatburn that rushes up the throat and fills the mouth with burning acid.

And this all indicates a bowel that is very unhappy.

It also indicates that all is not well with the immune system. And when someone has cancer, no matter what kind, that person needs the strongest immune defences they can possibly get.

Would you like some more proof that the bowel is an important part of the body's defence system?

Have you ever noticed something significant about children who get sick and are taken to the doctor? What does the doctor usually prescribe? Isn't it antibiotics?

And have you ever noticed something else. When a child has been on antibiotics they often seem to catch everything that's going around! They seem to be always in need of medical help.

And I have met children who have been on 'low grade' antibiotics for over a year. And they are not well kids.

The question I ask is this. 'Is it the disease that makes them sick or is it the constant antibiotics that makes them sick?'

Because, as you know, antibiotics are like mass murderers. They kill the good along with the bad. They don't think. They just go out like a hired gun and kill everything in sight. Boom, Boom, you're dead!

Sure, often this gets rid of the bad guys. But it also kills the good guys too. A bit like a movie where the good cop kills all the gangsters but goes on shooting until everyone at the scene is lying in a pool of blood.

So it should be obvious by now that the bowel is an

important part of the immune system.

It is not only antibiotics that upset the balance in the bowel. Stress, pollution, poor diet, too much sugar and so on, all play a part.

So what this means is that we have to boost the good guys in our bowel. Most people are aware of acidopholus but do not realise that there are different kinds of good bacteria along the bowel. And they all need reinforcing.

So a first step for anyone who has been on antibiotics is to take a course of good bowel bacteria. The bowel must be repopulated with good bacteria.

I believe everyone should take a course of bowel nutrients at least once a year, maybe even twice.

This was one of the first things I did when I discovered that I had a very aggressive prostate cancer.

It was a case of 'all hands to the pumps'. My ship of life was sinking and it was definitely a case of doing everything possible to save that ship.

And so I took a lot of bowel bacteria capsules.

My life was at stake. It was a fight with no holds barred.

And I desperately wanted to win.

And as I have said, the major job is to strengthen the body in every way possible so it can defend itself. Drugs weaken the body. They give the liver an extra task. The body has not only to fight the cancer, it now has the added burden of coping with the drugs too.

In my case, just the opposite of what I was trying to achieve.

THE TESTOSTERONE TRAP

I am a man. You are a man. And we both secrete testosterone. This is the male hormone… this is what makes us what we are!

And now I find testosterone is my enemy.

Turn to the next chapter and find out if we can do anything to defeat what was once our friend but is now our enemy!

6 Here are some things your doctor doesn't know about!

Whilst a lot of doctors like to give the impression they know everything about how to handle disease, they don't!

I can understand why they defend their image of 'all-knowing'.

It is very important if people are to get better that they believe in their doctor. It has been found time after time that where people trust their practitioner they tend to get better more quickly.

In the old days a doctor's 'bedside manner' was his most important asset. These days it is fashionable for the medical fraternity to mock the placebo effect. Which is what the 'bedside manner' was all about!

But years ago this was the doctor's most powerful weapon.

As you know, the placebo effect is where something is given to the patient that is inert, something that couldn't help the course of the disease.

And despite the pill being nothing but milk sugar, the patient gets better.

May I say, as an aside, that I don't really care what gets people better as long as they do get better. I can't see the point of knocking the placebo effect if it does the same thing as a drug, without the side effects.

When learned professors of medicine scoff at the placebo effect it reminds me of when I was at school. Some kids could get the right answers to mathematical problems by intuition.

The right answer popped into their minds just like that.

But the teacher would never accept it. There had to be proof. How did the student arrive at that answer? The teacher demanded to know how the answer was reached.

And the kid who had an intuitive grasp of mathematics couldn't tell the teacher how it happened. It just happened. And so he would not be given a mark even though he had the correct answer.

I wonder how many children had their mathematical genius snuffed out by teachers who didn't understand what was happening before their eyes.

And so why query the placebo effect? As long as it works, let's get on with it.

Let me give you another example of the placebo effect in action. Some years ago my best friend came to stay with Peg and I. We were delighted to welcome the whole family. Husband, wife and three girls and my friend's mother-in-law.

This lady was terrific. Not the mother-in-law of all the jokes. My friend really loved his mother-in-law. But when bedtime came... catastrophe.

She couldn't sleep without taking a sleeping pill and she had forgotten to bring them. No chance of getting any either. She needed a script to get some... no script. Too far from home to go and get some.

So I went into my clinic and brought out a little white tablet.

I told this lovely lady that this was the most powerful sleeping pill ever invented. I told her that I only gave people this sleeping tablet in dire emergencies. When all else had failed.

I told her not to take it until she was ready to get into bed because she could fall asleep on the stairs on the way up to her bedroom.

Next morning she came down radiant.

She told me she had had the best night's sleep she had had for years.

Then she asked me where she could get a supply of these wonder tablets. She expected me to tell her it was a herbal tablet containing secret herbs.

I had to confess it was a simple aspirin tablet given with strong suggestions. A placebo!

So I suggest that it doesn't do to scoff at things we may not fully understand. The main thing is that it helps the patient.

And so even though we understand why so many doctors want to appear infallible and therefore scoff at things they do not understand it doesn't make them correct.

As I have said before, your doctor is a caring person, doing his or her best within the confines of their training, there is a lot they don't know.

THE SPECIALIST SMILED WHEN I TOLD HIM WHAT I WAS GOING TO DO

The Urologist I saw for a second opinion is a very nice man. He is extremely competent at what he does as a well trained medical man.

He is also caring. He took time to explain everything about prostate cancer in general, and mine in particular. I learned a lot from him during our interviews.

But when I told him I was going to use all my talents as a Naturopath, Herbalist and Homeopath to fight the cancer he smiled. Bear in mind, my PSA was 126, horrifyingly high. His scepticism was understandable.

'Well, they won't do you any harm' was his comment.

Won't do you any harm can be interpreted as 'Can't do you any good either!'

But I was to prove him wrong!

They were going to do me a lot of good... and I hope the information I have discovered will do you a lot of good too.

I LEARN ALL ABOUT TESTOSTERONE...
WELL, ALMOST ALL

My friend, the Urologist, explained carefully that Testosterone was the problem. Testosterone, once the substance that made me male, was now killing me. From being on my side, testosterone was now out to get me.

He told me that my prostate was turning innocent testosterone into deadly dihydrotestosterone, called DHT for short. It is this DHT that turns into cancer.

He told me I had too much testosterone.

Now friend, I found this hard to understand.

Because as we men grow older our testosterone level goes down.

We find it harder to get sexually aroused. When at one time just looking at a centre-fold girl would get us excited, these days we would have to have the girl... and for quite a while before we finally got around to it!

A lot of men are so short of testosterone they can't keep an erection.

I mean, there are clinics that inject you with testosterone to revitalise the lagging libido!

And now I am told we men who have prostate problems have too much testosterone. It didn't make much sense to me.

I found it hard to believe that at 70 years of age I had too much testosterone.

Looking back, I had heaps of testosterone when I was younger. I was a swaggering, blustering, hard hitting testosterone-filled idiot. My whole mind seemed to be full of thoughts of beautiful girls — there was little room for anything else.

I had a hormonal rush in a big way. Overflowing testosterone!

But gradually things changed. As my testosterone levels went down my behaviour improved. I lost my macho image. I became more reasonable.

And now here was this man telling me I had too much testosterone.

Gosh, if I had too much I'd hate to be the guy with too little!

It didn't make sense to me.

However, I listened hard just the same. I needed to know all I could about prostate cancer… on the cancer Richter scale I was 8 out of 10. My testosterone, it seemed, was out of control.

The treatment seemed almost as bad as the disease!

So now we were going to get down to brass tacks. Take the gloves off and get into bare-knuckle facts.

And I didn't like what I heard.

There are a number of options all aimed at reducing the flow of testosterone to a trickle. Some aimed at stopping the tap altogether.

Now hold on to your seats as I go through the options facing me on that dreadful day.

The first is 'radical surgery'. I have met men who have had this done to them. One was an old friend. When we shook hands he couldn't look me in the face. He took my hand and turned his head away.

I couldn't understand why even when his lovely wife whispered he had had radical surgery for prostate cancer.

But now I found out that in radical surgery they cut off your testicles. The surgery nightmares are made of.

No wonder the poor man had a job to look me in the face. In his mind he had lost his manhood. He had paid what he considered a very high price to stay alive. And there are men who would rather be dead!

So that was one of the options. Stop the tap totally. Become an eunuch. The thought was terrifying.

'God, there has to be something else', I pleaded.

And there is.

Another option is to operate on the prostate itself. Cut out the cancer. Leave the healthy cells there. But I have learned that a lot of men who have this operation have bladder problems for the rest of their lives.

They leak all the time. They are incontinent. Like a baby. And far too many for my liking, just like a baby, have to wear a nappy.

Not a pleasant thought.

And even worse... quite often cutting away at the cancer seems to really annoy it. They don't get it all and it now becomes very belligerent. It goes on the attack. It jumps into other parts of the body and you now have cancer in another organ or tissue.

More nightmare material...

I was comforted when the Urologist told me he rarely operated on men over sixty. It was not a useful procedure at my age. So whilst I now knew about it, I wasn't going to have to endure it.

Thank God for small mercies, as they say.

The next option was drugs.

And the favourite among the physicians was the female hormone, estrogen.

They pump you full of this stuff and to all intents and purposes, you lose your male characteristics.

You can develop breasts like a female. God help me!

You would lose your male urges. I get the impression that once you are seventy the medicos don't think this is much of a hardship. How wrong can anyone be?

And in addition to the female hormone which is injected into you, there was another drug proposed. This one shut down my adrenal glands.

Now let me tell you, my friend, your adrenal glands are very important. The most obvious thing about them is that they pump out adrenaline. And it is adrenaline that gives you your get up and go.

People who are tired all the time often have what is called 'hypoadrenia'. Translated this means low adrenal output.

Adrenaline is the stuff that helps you cope with stress. Adrenaline is the stuff that helps you to run like a gazelle when some mugger demands your wallet.

When you hear about some little bloke doing things like Hercules, ripping off car doors when his wife is trapped inside and other remarkable feats, it is the adrenaline flooding his veins that gives him the power.

And now I was supposed to be happy about closing it down.

My thoughts were that I would now be a push-over for anyone who felt like bullying me. Instead of being a full-blooded male I would be a feminised version, without guts!

And there was more to come. When I am on this particular drug, it would be necessary to have a liver function test every month. Because this drug could cause me to have problems with my liver. And if this happened, I would need to have different drugs to deal with this situation.

It was all getting worse and worse.

It seemed that it was going to be downhill all the way from now on.

The next alternative was to do nothing.

To sit and wait to see if the cancer would leap somewhere else.

I was assured that this is often the preferred option.

Sit, watch, and do nothing. Presumably until it was too late to do anything. At least, that was my feeling about it.

It was explained to me that very often when men have this option they do not die from the prostate cancer.

No, they die from something else!

I could believe this if the patient was already in poor health.

Here are some things your doctor doesn't know about!

I know people who are on blood pressure drugs, blood thinning drugs, drugs for this and drugs for that. And in my opinion they are just as much on a life-support mechanism as someone plugged into the wall.

If you pull the plug out of the wall, the patient dies.

If you take away all the drugs, the patient also dies.

So under these circumstances it could well be the patient died from something else. Something he already had before the prostate cancer got hold of him.

But that wasn't the case with me.

I was as fit as the proverbial fiddle. I weight train three times a week. I still do, by the way. I was tested for cholesterol, below 4. Blood pressure of a twenty year old. Reflexes like a cat. Lungs like a track athlete.

Apart from the prostate cancer, the rest of me was in great shape.

So I was more likely to die from my prostate cancer than anything else. I didn't have anything else wrong with me!

So sitting and waiting and doing nothing was not an option for me.

The Urologist made out two prescriptions for me. One was for the injectable female hormone and the other for the adrenal drug.

These drugs have to go through the Health Commission first. The doctor just doesn't hand them to you 'over the counter'.

You finally get them in the mail some weeks later.

Then you go to your family doctor who takes over from then on.

You are also expected to go to your Urologist every six months or so for a check up.

After a lot of thought, I decided I would give the hormone drug a go but not the adrenal drug. I thought one was bad enough.

ARE MEDICAL RESEARCHERS ON THE WRONG TRACK?

All the efforts to help me survive were aimed at stopping the production of testosterone so it couldn't be converted into the deadly dihydrotestosterone.

But why not prevent the testosterone from being converted into the cancer-causing kind?

It seemed to me that all the research was focused on the wrong thing. The testosterone is not the bandit. It is whatever converts it into the DHT version. That is the real bandit. That is the enemy. That is where the effort should be focused.

Now there may be research going on in this direction. But if there is I haven't heard about it. Just looking for more powerful drugs.

The other options are radiation and chemotherapy.

But since I found out about my prostate cancer it is remarkable how many men I have met with prostate cancer.

And I have listened to a lot of horror stories.

And having radiation and chemo are not often pretty stories to listen to.

What horrified me was the result of the chemo and radiation.

I met one really pleasant man who had suffered having his testicles removed and radiation. He had a prolapsed stomach below the large slash across his belly where he had been opened up. And he had been told nothing could be done about it.

And whilst his PSA had gone down to safe levels he was now a sick man. He blames the operation and radiation for all his problems. He told me he felt quite well before it was discovered he had prostate cancer.

And now, whilst the cancer seems under control, his life is a misery.

Which reinforces my point that medical research should focus on stopping testosterone converting to the DHT.

So my goal now was to find out if there was any way possible to block off the converting of testosterone to DHT.

There had to be a way.

Of that I was confident.

But I now had to find it!

So I asked all the herbalists I know. I went through all the piles of articles, magazines, monograms and everything else I had stuffed into my files.

It was at this time I wished I had a better filing system.

Along the way I was becoming more and more knowledgeable about the prostate gland itself and about prostate cancer.

And I used myself as my own guinea pig. I used myself as the means of proving herbal and other non-drug substances could really help.

I desperately wanted to prove the medical view, that I was terminal, was wrong.

When you discover you have cancer and face death, Life itself becomes very precious.

Is this why so many men die of prostate cancer?

Prostate cancer kills as many men as breast cancer kills women.

But prostate cancer gets relatively little publicity. Compared to breast cancer, it is a non-starter. We see appeals to women to go and have their breasts examined regularly, don't we? When did you last see an advertisement of any kind telling men to go and have their prostate gland examined? Probably never!

And yet prostate cancer is the most common form of cancer in men. And only heart attacks kill more men than prostate cancer.

Just remember that at least 80% of men over 60 will get some form of prostate problem as they grow older. So you would think it would be considered pretty serious. But it seems like a secret disease.

Almost as though your average guy is ashamed to talk about it. And where cancer is concerned, ignorance is not bliss. It is asking for BIG trouble… big big trouble.

So it is essential, vital, that this problem be brought out into the open. Men must be educated to have regular check-ups, just like women for breast cancer.

In the case of prostate cancer, embarrassment kills!

Being either unwilling or unaware of the need to have regular check-ups can kill you. No messing about. Think about it.

A high price to pay for false modesty. Death is the ultimate penalty.

So your average guy goes on his merry way oblivious of the danger he is in. A bit like someone crossing the road totally unaware that a huge semi-trailer is boring down on him at 100 kilometres an hour!

Hopefully he will look up in time to jump out of the way but if he doesn't… SPLAT… he is all over the highway.

And we need more attention-grabbing methods to alert men to the danger they could be in.

And the other problem, in my opinion, is that most people are unaware of the options open should they be unlucky enough to find they have a prostate problem.

And that is the purpose of this book. I want you to know ALL the options open to you. Not just the medical ones. Only when you are in possession of ALL the facts can you really make an informed decision.

I am not writing this book to replace your doctor. Simply to inform you of the options open to help you with your problem.

It is my opinion that some men die needlessly. They die because the medical options ran out. But no-one realised that there are other options.

Options that could save lives!

My search for answers continued

It was not so long ago that we were told the human immune system could not be strengthened. It was illegal to advertise and say this or that product could boost the immune system.

But the facts were there. There are substances that do enhance the immune system. You can strengthen your bodily defences.

And the more I studied cancer in general and prostate cancer in particular, the more convinced I was that I was on the right path.

Have you ever seen a Herbal Pharmocopea? These are huge tomes, great heavy books packed with scientific information about herbs. It lists the contents of the herbs, relates each herb's medicinal values, the toxicity of any herbs, if any, exists. They are 'heavy' books for the average person to read.

But I had to find out all I could so I continued to wade through all this material and I want to share what I found with you. I want you to understand all the options open to you.

And in the next chapter I will reveal the first big discovery I made. There is a herb that blocks off the conversion of testosterone to DHT. There is a herb that everyone with prostate problems should be taking. And I feel it is important that I get this information to as many people as I can.

I want to get to the partners of men. Because quite often the partner is involved. It is not only the patient who will lose out should he die — his whole family and friends will be affected. Dramatically!

And it is partners who often persuade Mr Macho, Mr Embarrassed to have a digital examination — to go and be tested.

So I want everyone to know as much as possible about prostate cancer, the misery and the hopeful options.

Despair and apathy are your greatest enemies.

When men despair they fall into the pit of apathy. They are too far in the hole even to take their medicine. They are too deep in darkness to look for the light of knowledge that could save their life!

Winston Churchill, the great British World War II Statesman

said 'Never, never... NEVER give up!'

And he was right. I could have given up. I could have shared the alarm of the doctors when they found my PSA was 126. I could have slipped into the pit of despair when I found out that 60 percent of my prostate was cancerous.

In fact, as I related in the first two chapters, I started to slide down that slippery slope. I started to wallow in self-pity. I wanted to howl in despair. I was a voyeur masochistically watching my own funeral every night.

Fortunately, I woke up to myself.

Luckily I made the decision to DO something to help myself.

I made the choice to ignore the medicos. I made the choice to search for another way.

I remembered the old saying I was fond of quoting in my public speaking: 'If at first you don't succeed, TRY ANOTHER WAY'.

And the other way led away from drugs and the conventional treatments for prostate cancer.

Would you mind if I make a point that may not have a lot to do with treating the prostate gland but has a lot to do with being successful?

It is this.

How often do we as people ask ourselves if what we are doing is working for us?

Do we ever look at our behaviour to see if it is working for us?

The truth is boring people keep on boring. The same people keep going to jail. The same people keep losing everything on the horses or poker machines.

People in a relationship keep on destroying each other.

Nations keep going to war even though history tells us that war is a useless exercise that robs us of the flower of our youth.

Shouldn't we ask ourselves if there are other things we could be doing? If we are following one path and we are not getting better I have to ask the question 'Why do we keep on doing it?'

And the same thing applies to helping ourselves when we find we have prostate cancer.

Conventional treatment could simply be the same way of doing things even if they don't work. Remember I told you about Albert who was told he was terminal. He would die within the year!

Albert accepted that as a fact. Because he didn't examine the results of conventional treatment. He fell into the pit of despair and apathy. He was not prepared to look at the suggestion that there could be another way.

Remember, if at first you don't succeed (if conventional treatment is not working and the prognosis is you are a dead man), then try another way. Try the herbal way. Try the Homeopathic way. Try every way open to you.

Follow Churchill's advice. Never, never give up.

On paper Britain had no chance against the might of the German Forces massed against her. But the experts were wrong.

Britain triumphed over what seemed to be disaster.

And you too can triumph over disaster.

In the next chapter I will reveal to you the herb that blocks off DHT. Yes, there is a herb.

I want you to know about it.

7

On the road to recovery

I had felt the bony hand of the Grim Reaper on my shoulder. I had smelled the mould of the grave in my nostrils, I had felt the icy breath of Death on the back of my neck.

And it was horrible.

I wanted to feel the warmth of the sun on my back. I wanted the smell of roses and lavender in my nostrils. I wanted the hugs and kisses of my family. I wanted to see my grandchildren grow up.

I wanted LIFE!

And that spurred me on.

When I had got over the shock of finding I had terminal cancer, I was determined to beat it in six months.

This is known as 'breakthrough' goal setting. It was first formally used in the computer industry. What you do is set yourself what seems to be an impossible goal. A goal that others think cannot possibly be reached.

And then you set about finding ways to make it happen!

To set myself the goal of beating cancer in

six months in the face of expert medical opinion could be considered a bit of an impossible goal.

But only if you accept that medical opinion is infallible. And it isn't. I was once told that even at the most sophisticated American medical faculty, they were wrong in their diagnosis 50% of the time.

So there was room to move.

And in the great book *You Can't Afford The Luxury Of A Negative Thought* the author advises: 'In the case of terminal disease concentrate on those that do survive. If out of 10,000 diagnosed cases, 1,000 survive... focus your attention on the 1,000, NOT on the 9,000 who don't make it'.

And I found that good advice. If 1,000 could survive then so could I. Especially as I had more knowledge than the average cancer patient.

I was lucky. I did not rely on cancer experts for all my advice.

AND SO NOW I HAD TO MAKE THE SIX-MONTH CURE GOAL HAPPEN

As I said earlier, I believe a lot of research should go into stopping testosterone converting to the deadly dihydrotesterone.

And I found that there is a lot of herbal knowledge in this area.

Prostate problems have been around a very long time. Thousands of years. And so have herbs!

So the first area I decided to look was in herbals.

And there is a herb used a lot by Herbalists for this very purpose and it is called Saw Palmetto. It is also known as Sabal Serrulata.

And it is freely available in any Health Food Store.

It is a major ingredient in any herbal formula for the prostate.

HERBS ARE NOT OLD WIVES TALES

The medical establishment would have you believe that there is no firm scientific evidence for the use of botanical medicines. This is not true.

Let me tell you that doctors prescribed aspirin for years. But did you know that the main mechanism of action responsible for aspirin's anti-inflammatory effect was not known until the early 1970s! And how aspirin controls pain is still not fully understood. But this doesn't stop doctors from prescribing aspirin. Nor should it!

You will be interested to learn that 25% of all prescription drugs contain active constituents obtained from plants.

But ingrained prejudice is hard to overcome.

Listen to this for a moment. Syphilis first came to Europe from the West Indies — this was in 1574. The physicians of the day reasoned that diseases native to a particular country could be cured with herbs from that same country.

You can imagine the outcry if that was suggested to medical people today. Quackery! (The favourite cry of the uninformed medical mind.)

Regardless of this a French physician called Nicolas Mondardes investigated the herb Sarsaparilla. And guess what, he found it was very effective in treating syphilis.

Sarsaparilla was also used by the Chinese to treat syphilis. Blood tests revealed that Sarsaparilla was effective in 90% of cases treated!

In 1812 during the Napoleonic Wars in Portugal it was discovered that Portugese soldiers who were treated with Sarsaparilla recovered much faster than the British soldiers, who were treated with mercury.

It baffles the intelligence to discover that although sarsaparilla was quite clearly a more effective method of treating this disease, mercury became the standard treatment of the day.

It has since been discovered that what once was thought to be tertiary syphilis was really mercury poisoning.

I tell you this to reassure you that using herbs to help with prostate cancer or preventing it is a well researched way.

For an enlarged prostate, herbs should be your treatment of choice.

And certainly for prostate cancer I believe sincerely that there are herbs you should be making as part of your total programme to restore health.

To achieve my 'breakthrough' goal I was determined to use everything I could lay my hands on that would help me.

I have spoken with a lot of men with prostate problems and I can tell you that very few indeed knew anything about herbs to help them.

Which reminds me of some advice I was given years ago by a very successful man. He said to me 'Ron, look at what everyone else is doing… **and don't do it**!' His reasoning was that most people are sadly unsuccessful in most areas of their lives. The conclusion he came to was that what they were doing was not working for them. And if it wouldn't work for them, it wouldn't work for him either.

So if most people with prostate problems know nothing about herbs and rely on drugs, I decided I would look for my answers elsewhere.

I researched Saw Palmetto… and this is what I found out

First up, Saw Palmetto is really a berry used like a herb. No matter what they call it… herb, berry… it doesn't matter. What it does is what matters.

Saw Palmetto is also known as *Sabal Serrulata*. *Serenoa repens* or *Serenoa serrulata*. You need to know this in case you are looking at Saw Palmetto under one of its other names and don't realise it is what you want.

Saw Palmetto definitely inhibits the conversion of testosterone to the most undesirable dihydrotestosterone. It blocks the attachment of DHS to cellular binding sites. It also does something else very useful and desirable. It increases the breakdown and excretion of DHS.

Which is just what I wanted, and so do you!

This is not folklore. It is not an 'old wives tale', it is not quackery.

No, my friend, it is cold hard facts. Backed up by over 20 double-blind placebo controlled tests.

It is a *scientific* fact that Saw Palmetto is one of the master herbs when it comes to doing something about an enlarged or diseased prostate.

What is more, Saw Palmetto has been shown to reduce the pain and inflammation of an enlarged prostate.

So you have more than one reason to embrace Saw Palmetto.

If you don't want an enlarged prostate (and remember something like 80% of men over 60 have one!) or you have something more serious as I did, put Saw Palmetto at the head of your list of remedies.

And what is beautiful about it is you can get it in any good Health Food Store and it has no known side effects. Which is more than you can say for the drugs used!

How the humble evening primrose flower helps

In my research for herbs to help me achieve my goal I discovered that men with enlarged prostate glands usually exhibit elevated levels of a substance called Prostaglandin E2.

What is a Prostaglandin?

Simplified, it is a sort of hormone that sits in the tissue. It doesn't wander around like a key looking for lock-like 'ordinary' hormones.

And it so happens that Prostaglandin E2 causes inflammation. In the case of the prostate it can be severe inflammation causing considerable pain.

Now here is something very interesting. The oil of the seeds from the Evening Primrose contains a good amount of a Prostaglandin.

But it is a Prostaglandin that knocks the E2 type on the head. That means it **reduces** inflammation!

So yippee! There is another natural substance that could help me.

Why you need essential fatty acids to win

Evening Primrose Oil also contains what is called Omega 6. And Omega 6 is what is called an 'essential fatty acid'.

So what on earth is an essential fatty acid. At first glance you could be forgiven for exclaiming who wants more fat and who wants acid?

Well, despite its name it is neither of those things.

There are two essential fatty acids that I believe help. The Omega 6 from Evening Primrose Oil and the Omega 3 from deep sea fish or Flaxseed.

Research has shown that men with prostate problems are often low in both these Omega's

By the way, the word 'essential' when referring to these fatty acids means your body cannot produce them. You have to get them from outside your body.

I found a very good combination of Omega 3 and Omega 5 in one capsule. So I started taking one of these three times a day.

As most people are low in these and most people don't take them (because they don't know about them) it was a good reason to take them.

A further illustration of watch what everyone else is doing and don't do it. If most men with prostate problems are low in these essential fatty acids it is an excellent reason to take them!

I believed I was hot on the trail now and my confidence that I would achieve my six-month goal increased.

THE HIDDEN POWER OF EPILOBIUM

In 1986 an Austrian lady called Maria Treben published a book called *Health From God's Garden*. This book became an international best-seller. The sub-title of the book is 'Herbal Remedies for Glowing Health and Glorious Well-Being'. Quite a promise.

In this book Maria Treben mentions Epilobium or 'Small Flowered Hairy Willow Herb'. A lot of people latch on to the word 'willow' and think the herb comes from a special kind of willow tree. In fact, I have heard people ask for small leaf willow tree tea.

But Epilobium does not come from a tree. It really has no connection at all with weeping willows or any other kind of willow tree.

It is, in fact, a herb.

It is a sad fact but most of the time we humans walk through this wonderful earth totally blind to its wonders. Instead of seeing healing herbs put there to help us, we see only weeds. Instead of rain forests we see unmade profits, and chop them down.

I wonder how many magical herbs possessed of unimaginable healing power we have blindly destroyed by cutting down or burning millions of hectares of 'jungle'?

We have managed to save a few herbs with incredible powers, Gurarana is one and one I will go into greater depth later, Cat's Claw.

But we were just lucky to salvage these.

We have to wake up and actually observe the world around us.

Tell you what, finding out you have cancer certainly sharpens the senses and makes one really appreciate every breath. The world takes on new meaning. Everything is a pleasure.

And you realise the stupidity of letting little things interfere with your pleasure in just being alive.

Anyway, getting back to the small-flowered hairy willow herb.

There is more than one variety of this herb. There is a great hairy willow herb with big flowers. But the one we are interested in has small white to deep pink flowers. It is not a conspicuous herb. In fact, if it were a human being you would pass it in a crowd without noticing it.

And just as you could pass someone with incredible powers in a crowd without realising who you were passing, so you would pass the small flowered willow herb.

But this herb has a particular affinity for the prostate gland.

Have you ever thought how almost magical it is that certain herbs have an affinity with very definite human organs or body systems?

Dandelion, Celandine, Blue Flag — these are all 'liver' herbs. Uva Ursi, Juniper are urinary tract herbs. And as I go through the herbal Pharmacopea I am amazed how the herbs all have properties beneficial to mankind.

I find it hard to believe that this world was created just by chance. Everything smacks of a superior intelligence. As someone once remarked 'If this world, this universe is just an act of chance, then a hurricane blowing through a junkyard should be able to construct a Boeing 747!'

Perhaps we humans are too arrogant. We think we can conquer Nature... But the first cyclone, the first floods, the first earthquakes, the first famines should remind us of who is **really** in charge here!

And somehow, sitting there is the small-flowered willow herb. An inconspicuous weed to many. But a botanical miracle to others.

And it is a wonderful herb for helping the prostate gland. It is a specific for the prostate. There are many men who used to get up umpteen times through the night to empty their bladder. Standing there waiting for the flow to start. Watching the dribble instead of the full forced flow. And a little later having to go again because the enlarged prostate was stopping the bladder from emptying properly. A miserable existence.

It is at times like these that a man wonders what happened to him. Where did his strength go to? Is this what aging is all about?

But those men who have taken small-leaf willow tea or taken capsules or a liquid are blessing the day. Now they don't get up anything like they used to. And the flow is a lot stronger.

And if this is not magic, then I wonder what is.

So add Epilobium to your list of herbs. I take it in a tincture.

My reason is that I had prostate cancer and I believed I needed my herbs in stronger doses than someone with simply an enlarged prostate.

I urge any man over 40 who is reading this book to drink Epilobium tea every day. This way you will avoid the anquish I wrote about in the first two chapters of this book! And that alone will show you a profit a hundred times greater than the money you paid for this book!

FAMOUS CHINESE HERB TO THE RESCUE

When you mention the word 'ginseng' a lot of men give a knowing look. 'Ah, yes, Ginseng. Isn't that some kind of aphrodisiac? Kind of stimulates sexual ability or desire or something, doesn't it?'

The truth is that neither the ancient Chinese nor the modern ones see Ginseng as an aphrodisiac. They see it as a tonic herb.

And an especially good tonic herb for the male endocrine system.

Ginseng takes time to work. You cannot expect a 'quick fix' with Ginseng. You must take it for several months.

People often ask me how soon they can expect results when they have decided to take herbs or other supplements. And they are usually disappointed with my answer.

The truth is we are all biologically individual. We don't all digest our food as efficiently as others. Our stomachs are not all the same size. We don't have exactly the same colons. Some are very poor and others are good. We don't feel, think, act the same.

And so we will all react differently not only to medication of whatever kind, but we all react differently to disease. Look at influenza as an example. Some people get feverish and are hot and sweaty. Others get feverish and are dry and hot. Some get aching bones. Some get a cough. But when you look at it, very few people have exactly the same reaction to the flu virus.

And it is the same with medication.

When I was injected with Zoladex I broke out in the most horrendous rash all over my back and arms. It looked and felt horrible. But not everyone who has Zoladex reacts like that.

I believe I did because I am relatively healthy. My body was doing its best to throw out the drug through my skin. My body didn't like the drug and was giving me a clear message.

Mind you, when you first discover you have cancer you find it everywhere. It is like being afraid of a boogieman — you find them in every dark closet, you suspect they are waiting to leap out on you with ravening fangs and claws.

So it is with cancer. When I saw the rash my first horrified thought was that I had got melanoma. It's funny how common sense deserts a person in a crisis.

My doctor unwittingly made things worse. He suspected the drug had made me photosensitive. I was now sensitive to sunlight. He gave me a prescription, which I threw in the bin! It was simply a bad reaction to the drug.

I tell you this so you will understand we are not all the same. We all have different reactions to herbs and supplements. So if it isn't working as fast as you would like, be patient. Because, my friend, even though you may not be aware of it, things are changing for the better inside your body. Believe me!

Ginseng is what is called an 'adaptogen'. This means it restores balance in the body. When we are sick we are out of balance. So restoring balance is an essential part of any treatment programme.

Ginseng is called *Jenshen* in China where it is commonly used for impotence. If Ginseng helps impotence, and there is a lot of anecdotal evidence to say it does, it is because it is a tonic for the male sexual system.

The Chinese insist that Ginseng does not stimulate the glands into unnatural activity. It is seen as a **restorer** of the sexual system. A team of Soviet scientists confirmed the power of Ginseng, They established that the root does have a beneficial effect on the male sexual organs and other glands. The Doctor in charge of the research said that Ginseng acts only by improving physiological processes. No bad effects are observed after taking it.

It is important that you buy only the best quality ginseng. Cheap Ginseng could hardly have the same medicinal properties as the top varieties.

Be aware of the difference between Panax Ginseng and Siberian Ginseng. They are not the same thing.

It is Panax Ginseng I am talking about here. Most Panax these days seems to come from Korea. The Government controls the cultivation of Ginseng and the quality is indicated on the packet. They have different qualities, usually in different coloured packing.

Siberian Ginseng is to Ginseng as an onion is to garlic. Related, but not the same. Siberian Ginseng came to fame in the 1972 Olympics when it was publicised as the 'Russian Secret Weapon'.

At those Olympics the Russian athletes carried all before them. Their training and nutrition was a closely guarded secret. That was in the days of the so-called 'iron curtain'. Eventually, it leaked out that their athletes were all given Siberian Ginseng as part of their training programme.

As a result there was a boom in the sales of Siberian Ginseng, as you would expect. So Siberian Ginseng is good for energy but you want Panax Ginseng, the best quality you can get.

How a humble weed can help you

Clover is seen as a curse in a lot of lawns but it can be a life-saver for someone with a prostate problem.

Clover contains what are known as 'phytestrogens'. This means estrogen from plants.

However, research has shown that clover helps normalise sex hormones in men as well as women. From a prostate cancer viewpoint, taking Red Clover as a source of estrogen seems a better bet than having female hormones injected.

But Red Clover contains something else! Something special.

It contains something called Geniston. And do you know what Geniston does? It chokes off the blood supply to the cancer cells.

You may remember I said that cancer cells demand more and more blood. They even create their own vascular system to feed themselves.

Self-perpetuating little Draculas. They want blood and more blood.

But Genisten helps to shut down the blood supply. And this starves the cancer cells. And starved cancer cells cannot carry on their deadly work.

So I added Red Clover to the herbs I take. And the results speak for themselves.

Red Clover is sold in most Health and Nutrition Centres. But they sell it for females. They sell it for menopause. But most will not know there is a powerful reason for someone with cancer to take it.

Who would believe that the humble clover in your lawn has such powerful properties. And people put weedkiller on it.

On March 17th every year clover becomes a Shamrock and now you know about Genisten all clovers are secretly four-leaf clovers!

Definitely something to put on your list!

ANOTHER LIFE-SAVING HERB FROM THE JUNGLE

Vast areas of the jungles of South America and Asia are being bulldozed every day. Once great tracts of jungle, they are now poor pasture land for beef cattle.

And who knows what botanical treasures have been destroyed in the process? It could be that a cure for AIDS has been trampled under the grinding tread of the bulldozers. Maybe a cure for melanoma has been thoughtlessly destroyed.

We could easily have allowed a treasure chest of botanical medicine to be lost forever. These herbs were placed there for our benefit, but like spoiled children we have carelessly thrown them away.

This should be of great concern to us all. Governments or should I rather say, politicians, don't seem concerned. After all, they don't think there are many votes in sincerely taking steps to save our planet.

But they and we should be.

As a matter of interest, we hear a lot about global warming. The increase of carbon dioxide in the atmosphere. We rightly lay a lot of blame at the doors of car exhaust and industry.

But the greatest source of oxygen, the greatest burners of excess carbon dioxide were the rain forests of the world. And these are being destroyed at a rate that is hard to believe.

And we will pay for it in due course. For every action there is an opposite reaction. Push and shove. Bound and rebound. Up and Down. In and out… and so it goes!

A SOUTH AMERICAN JUNGLE HERB TO THE RESCUE

Fortunately, one herb has been discovered before being destroyed. And thank heavens for that! It is called CAT'S CLAW.

Its botanical name is *Uno de Gata*, so you could find it under either name.

And Cat's Claw is a wonderful herb, believe me.

It is really a vine and gets its name from the way it entwines itself up the towering trees of the jungle. It has thousands of little hooks like claws that it uses to attach itself to the tree.

The South American Indians thought these hooks looked like cat's claw so that is how it got its name — *Uno de Gata*, Claw of the Cat.

Medical Convention praises Cat's Claw

At a medical convention in Lima, Peru, over 80 speakers praised the herb Cat's Claw. The claims made for this herb were remarkable.

Different specialists stood up in front of their peers and read out the results of their scientific studies on Cat's Claw.

The Scientists told how they had helped arthritis with Cat's Claw.

And most important from our point of view, how they had helped people with cancer. Even those whose cancers were considered to be inoperable. So hope was given to the medically hopeless!

As a result of all the work being done on the benefits of Cat's Claw, this herb is the biggest selling herb in North America. And what is more, it is now being imported by the **ton** into Europe.

It is predicted that Cat's Claw will soon be the biggest selling herb in the whole world within a few years.

And this is because the evidence says it works.

I take Cat's Claw every day as part of my 'Beat Cancer' regime.

And it would be a good idea to make it part of yours too.

Put the odds in YOUR favour!

My whole purpose as a Naturopath when helping people with cancer of any kind is to put the odds in their favour.

When people discover the horrible fact that they have cancer they are at their most vulnerable. At that stage they are most easily manipulated. Reason goes out of the window chased out by fear!

And that is normal and natural.

Unfortunately, most conventional cancer treatment tends to put the odds against the patient. His or her body is already battling an enemy. While some drugs are necessary all drugs throw an additional burden on the body.

The cancer patient's mental attitude also tends to work against him or her. They are tested, prodded, pushed and have all sorts of things done to them.

As I have remarked previously, they get the attitude of a victim.

But once the patients start doing things for themselves, their attitudes subtly change. They feel they are taking charge of their lives again.

I believe this is an essential part of the healing process.

We have to stop being a victim and take charge.

When we establish a regime of diet, vitamin, herb and supplements we are doing something positive. We are influencing the outcome ourselves.

We are busily putting the odds back in our favour.

We are ridding the body of accumulated toxins. We are giving our body the ammunition, the extra battalions it needs to overcome the enemy.

Doesn't this make a lot of sense to you?

It's a funny thing. When I lay out a regime for patients, even those with very serious illness, they will often say 'If I take all those I'll rattle!'

As though they are an empty gourd with a few dried beans rattling around inside. I point out that they don't say that about the different drugs they take. Some patients cheerfully take heart tablets, blood thinning tablets, high blood pressure tablets, fluid reducing tablets… they have their breakfast and then have a second breakfast of drugs.

And they don't protest that these will make them 'rattle'.

It seems only herbs and other supplements have this ability.

Of course, it is a lot of rubbish. People don't think they will 'rattle' if they have another helping of spinach pie, or another dollop of ice cream.

Herbs and supplements are not drugs per se. They are supplements. Supplements to your daily diet.

So when you lay out your own anti-cancer regime do what I do.

As I down my tablets, capsules or liquids I murmur: 'Terrific… another lot of extra-strength cancer killers'. And so I reinforce the good effect of the herb by washing it down with a good helping of positive suggestion.

It worked for me and I am sure it will work for you.

You CAN do it. Yes you can. What one person has done so can another. If I could beat cancer, my honest and fervent belief is that you can too.

Let me remind you again of breakthrough goal setting.

First set the impossible goal. For me it was to beat terminal prostate cancer in six months. Impossible according to the most expert of authorities.

Then search for ways to make it happen.

Well, let's set that same goal for you.

And in this book you will find information to help you get there!

Just DO IT! And keep on doing it.

In the next chapter let's look at ways to bring enormous extra power to your bodily defence system.

8 | God is on the side of the big battalions

A common custom during a war is to get the man of the Church to bless the guns. To invoke God's help in the struggle ahead with the enemy.

One dictator was famous for his comment 'God is on the side of the big battalions'. He meant that the general with the most troops and the most effective weaponry would win regardless of any blessing bestowed by the Church.

I put a different meaning on it.

God, the Cosmic Mind, the Universal Intelligence, call it what you will, is better able to help someone with the 'big battalions'.

In this case, the big battalions are the supplements fed to your body to give vital help in its battle against cancer.

So let us discuss ways to turbocharge your immune system doing the things I have done and still do!

BUT FIRST... WHY SHOULD YOU SUPERCHARGE YOUR IMMUNE SYSTEM?

Why do you need a super immune system?

Because your life depends on it!

In fiction we see Superman — he leaps across mighty rivers and jumps over tall buildings in one bound. But in real life we need an immune system capable of overwhelming any opposition. We need an immune system that puts the fear of God in any cancer cells or other 'nasties' that invade our body.

As soon as these foreign agents enter our body we need an immune system that can launch an immediate and overwhelming attack. We need an immune system 'blitzkrieg'. We need an immune system that can devastate any virus, germ or mutant cell that shows up in the body.

But most people don't have one!

Oh sure, most people have a day-to-day immune system.

They manage to fight off a fair amount of attack, colds and things like that. But should influenza rear its ugly head, down they go. Some people seem to catch everything that's going. A sure sign of a deficient immune system. And then there are all those people who have been on antibiotics of one kind or another, their immune system is almost certain to be down.

But to protect yourself against an enemy with all the trappings of cancer, you need an immune system built like a battle ship.

How narrow is your comfort zone?

Can I digress for a moment?

When we are talking about beating cancer in six months or preventing cancer even though your family is full of it, there would be a certain amount of disbelief.

While you hope what I am telling you is true, a little voice whispers in your ear. I mentioned this voice before when talking about affirmations. It is the same voice that limits you in all areas of your life.

This little voice says things like 'Mmm, it's OK for someone like him, he's a Naturopath' or 'What a load of malarky, does he expect me to do all this?' And so on and so on.

It's the same when we are called to do something out of the general run of experience. Something holds us back. We are tied with invisible ropes that lock us into the safe, the familiar.

Let me give you an example.

In a survey in America it was found that the average person is afraid of various things. Spiders, for example, are high on most peoples' list of things they hate. So are snakes of any kind.

But do you know the greatest dread people have?

It's the fear of standing up in public and giving a speech. That fear was greater than the fear of dealing with a large spider or a venomous snake.

Why would that be?

Because standing up there all exposed generates indescribable terror.

It means moving out of our comfort zone. Our comfort zone is where we feel safe. Where we like to be best in all the world.

It is our comfort zone that stops us joining a party. It stops us from chatting to strangers. It stops us from trying new foods or going to new places. As far as men are concerned, it stops us asking the way when we can't find our way. That's a fact, by the way, women have no problem asking for advice, but men do have a problem.

In fact, it is our comfort zone that limits our growth. It is the comfort zone influence that fosters the attitude 'nothing should be done for the first time'. Or the other block to progress, 'Not invented here'.

It is the comfort zone that colours our view of people of a different race or culture. It is the comfort zone that makes people herd together with people of the same interests. The worst example being crime gangs.

Better to be in a gang than out there on your own!

So to beat the stuffing out of cancer, or to stop cancer getting its filthy claws on you, you have to be prepared to move out of your comfort zone.

What's this got to do with herbs and stuff?

What has this got to do with herbs and stuff? A lot.

For me taking all these things is not a problem. After all, I have been a Naturopath for almost twenty years. I prescribe these things for various complaints every day. I have taken vitamins as a matter of course for years.

But for you it could be a very different matter.

For most all of your life you have been involved with doctors. If you are feeling off or are sick, where do you go? Naturally, to your doctor.

And what do you get? Good old familiar drugs. Antibiotics, cortisone, warfarin, blood pressure pills and so on. And they all have their place in restoring people to health.

The comfort zone, for a lot of people when they are sick, is a doctor.

Because that is what we are trained to do.

That's probably what our Mum and Dad do. It is what our brothers and sisters do. So do our friends.

So taking the advice of a Naturopath, taking lots of herbs and supplements is a whole new ball game.

And it can be uncomfortable.

It requires courage to move out of our comfort zone.

When I taught public speaking my biggest hurdle was to get people out of their comfort zone. That is staying safe with the bottom on a chair. Have you noticed at meetings people are very vocal if they are sitting down or among a crowd?

That's because they are anonymous. They are safe. Ask that same person to come up on the platform and repeat their message and they are immediately rendered speechless. If they do get up there they stumble or lose the thread of what they want to say. They sweat heavily too. Their stomach churns.

And all because they have moved out of their comfort zone.

But for you to beat cancer or make sure you don't get it, you will have to move out of your comfort zone.

WHAT WILL THEY THINK ABOUT ME?

It is surprising really, how we as adults are so afraid of what 'they' might say or think about us. Think about walking down the street in clothes that you don't usually wear. If you are very conservative in your taste, imagine walking down your street in just a pair of swimming briefs. Ugh, not the best of feelings. I mean, what would the neighbours think?

This even extends to things like the car we buy. And this works two ways. If you live in an up-market residential area where most people drive Jaguars and Mercedes, you would be reluctant to drive in a beat-up second-hand bomb. I mean, what would the neighbours think?

You could find yourself socially unacceptable!

And what if you live in a poor neighbourhood where most people do drive second-hand bombs? You pitch up in your new Mercedes and what will probably happen? Your neighbours' kids will be likely to take the wheels off. At least they will scratch your paintwork with a coin.

Because in both cases, not only are you out of your comfort zone, you have placed your neighbours outside their comfort zone too.

But if you are to win the cancer war, you will be called to move out of your comfort zone quite a few times. Your beliefs are being challenged. You have to face criticism for buying and taking supplements outside your normal run of life.

But YOU CAN DO IT!

You have in you tremendous powers you have never harnessed. You have the power to do almost anything you choose. Remember what I said about 'breakthrough' goal setting?

Just to set a compelling breakthrough goal requires you to move out of your comfort zone.

So remember, if you feel uncomfortable about doing or thinking about something, it is your comfort zone tugging at you and it means you should ignore it and push on.

Break through the barriers erected by your comfort zone.

Smash through into a world of light, beauty and accomplishment.

Once you leave the debris of your comfort zone behind you, your life will change. You will fly like an eagle. And won't that be wonderful?

Because then anything becomes possible.

Your colon is the heart of your immune system

People die slowly every day because of poor colon health!

Every single day.

And that is a needless tragedy.

Antibiotics, unbalanced diet, stress — all take their toll.

We normally think of our colon as a garbage disposal system. It's where the waste goes after we have digested our food. We know the colon is 'down there', but we don't know much else about it.

People often come to me and complain they have 'stomach ache'. Only one thing though, they are usually clutching the colon area and not the stomach!

But your colon is much more than a waste disposal system.

Your ability to defend yourself against the nasties that would ruin your life depends more than you think on your colon.

The ultimate in an unhealthy colon is colon cancer. And that is one of the fastest growing cancer problems in the modern world. That is, after prostate cancer!

My father was a fanatic about colon cleanliness. He believed that to have a healthy colon, it had to be scoured clean to be free of 'germs'. And to that end he drank strong concoctions of senna pods and other purgatives.

And he was totally wrong!

A healthy colon is not antiseptically 'clean'. It is a hotbed of germs. There are all sorts of germs in the bowel. Good and bad.

This idea of scouring the colon to get it 'clean' is not only wrong, it is downright dangerous. My father got bowel cancer and I believe it was because of his obsession with colon 'health'.

THE PROBLEM IS THE MIX OF BACTERIA IN THE COLON

The problem is with the kind of bacteria in the bowel. A lot of problems arise because the bowel is overpopulated with bad guys.

Antibiotics kill germs. The trouble is they kill indiscriminately. Good and bad bacteria are slaughtered. And the crafty bad bacteria seem much more able to re-colonise than the good guys. So the bowel gets an overabundance of bad bacteria.

That is why I recommend to all my patients that they take a good multi-acidopholus capsule after being on antibiotics. I sugggest they get an acidopholus complex. That is a capsule with about eight different kinds of bacteria in it. Take a whole course of these capsules.

The idea is to overwhelm the bad guys. To have a colon populated with lots of healthy bacteria.

Did you know that bacteria in your bowel manufacture Vitamin B? Yes, they do that and more. They are all part of your immune system.

You will notice that when a child has been on antibiotics, they seem to catch everything going. And so do adults.

This is not to say that antibiotics should not be prescribed. That would be a nonsense thing to say. But I do think they are prescribed carelessly.

It seems to me lazy medicine to give antibiotics for everything from cuts and scratches to the flu. Especially as antibiotics don't work on the flu. This is because influenza is caused by a virus. And antibiotics don't touch viruses.

Often, if questioned, a doctor will glibly say he is giving the antibiotics 'in case there is a secondary infection'. Well, let us cut off a woman's breasts in case she gets breast cancer, Let us cut out a man's prostate gland when he is young so he won't get prostate cancer as he ages. Let's give people antibiotics every day in case they get something or other.

It is unwise to take antibiotics unless you really need them.

The emergence of 'super bugs', bacteria immune to our strongest antibiotics should strike terror in all our hearts.

The day can come when we have no answer to attacks from deadly germs. If you get the flu, you die. If you have an operation and get septic, you die. Tuberculosis will kill you. There could easily be mass epidemics that sweep the globe. Epidemics that make the Black Death seem like a teddy bear's picnic.

This is the grim reality facing humanity today. It is not science fiction, it is a real threat. And micro-biologists all round the world are very concerned and so should we.

It seems that a major problem with people taking antibiotics for everything is that it depresses your natural defences.

Imagine a country that has a strong defence force. A well trained army equipped with the latest in modern weaponry. A highly mobile force that could bring overwhelming might to bear in any threatening situation. A defence force so formidable that enemies could be detected immediately they landed. And a defence force so well equipped that a powerful fighting force could arrive and attack the invader almost before they could hit the beach.

Now imagine you have a Government who decides to 'privatise' this fighting force by farming out the job of defending the country to private enterprise.

Well, the first thing that would happen is the contractors would reduce the number of fighting men. They would tell you that with modern equipment we don't need all those men. Then they would do an inventory of the equipment. They would stop buying weaponry because it was too expensive and reduced profits.

Very soon the country would end up with a second-rate defence force. Costs would be cut. The politicians would point to the savings on the balance of payments and so on.

But that country would now have an inferior force.

When invaders arrived they would not be detected so quickly. The defending troops would take longer to get there. The invaders would have time to get 'dug in'.

And the members of the original fighting force have already left. The up-to-the-minute weaponry has deteriorated. Instead of a world-class fighting force, you now have a second-rate one.

And it is the same with the body!

Your natural immune system is the top fighting force

Your own immune system, if intact, is like the superior fighting force. After years of indiscriminate taking of antibiotics, your natural defence system is weakened.

It is like the army that has been 'privatised'. It can no longer do a good job for you. Now, whenever your body is attacked, you seem unable to shake off the sickness. They take longer and hit harder.

And so you resort to more antibiotics.

And this makes your problem worse!

It is in your own interests to take charge of your bowel. Take charge of the job of boosting your natural defence force. You are the general. You are the boss.

Get your defence force back where it can do lightning strikes on any invader attacking your body. A tough, two-fisted, hard hitting, block-busting defence system.

A healthy defence system takes care of cancer everyday. Autopsies have revealed people had scar tissue in their lungs from cancer that was unable to take hold. There is ample evidence to show how our bodies deal with cancer and other aberrant cells every day. It's true!

That is why I tell people who have cancer that the major task is to boost the health of the 'host'. Give our body all the help it needs to not only defend us but to also beat the heck out of the cancer cells.

And you can do this. I did it and so can you.

I keep repeating this message right through this book. I want you to BELIEVE the truth, you CAN beat the cancer. No matter how gloomy the doctors may be.

Can I digress yet again?

It is important.

When your doctor or specialist looks at you over his spectacles and intones gravely 'I am very sorry, Mr Jones, but there is nothing more we can do for you. I suggest you take the *Capri Option*. That is, go home, get your affairs in order and enjoy yourself, as far as you can, for the next few months until you die'.

Some option!

And he is right. There is nothing more that can be done for you. But only speaking medically. Only if you are referring to drugs. But this well-meaning medical man knows nothing about Homeopathy. He knows nothing about Herbal Medicine. He knows nothing about using vitamins and other supplements therapeutically. He usually only know drugs and surgery, chemo and radiation.

And what is worse. Often that is all he **wants** to know! I sometimes get the impression that the doctor would be upset if his diagnosis was proved incorrect.

He would not say it was great that herbs did a job he couldn't do.

No, he would protest that there must have been a wrong diagnosis. Or the other great excuse, the disease must have gone into 'spontaneous remission'. Brilliant! But no credit for anything else that may have taken place.

And this attitude can be dangerous for your health!

Let me take a minute of your time to tell you a true story.

Many years ago I had a patient with cancer. As ever, not being allowed to treat cancer (it is a medical monopoly), I was giving support. The patient was doing well on Homeopathy and supplements.

Suddenly, I stopped seeing this patient. About six months later his wife came by and I enquired after her husband as I hadn't seen him for months.

Then she told me this horrible story.

It seems the local Community Nurse came by and saw his bottles of Homeopathic medicine and the supplements. Her reaction reeked of medical prejudice. This is what she said...

'What's that garbage you have there!'

When told it was medicine from a Naturopath this is what she said...

'You'd better get rid of that garbage **or the specialist won't treat you**.'

This blackmail caused him to go back solely on to drugs and he died. He paid a high price for her prejudice. And she knew absolutely nothing about Homeopathy or herbs or anything else outside her own medical background.

But it didn't stop her using blackmail to get the patient off anything else but drugs.

And I have no doubt that her response to boosting the colon as part of an immune system strengthening exercise would meet with equal prejudice. By the way, I believe that the word 'prejudice' is another word for IGNORANCE.

What you eat strengthens or weakens your immune system

A major reason why so many people get sick these days is malnutrition. Malnutrition means bad nutrition. Or perhaps, uninformed nutrition would be a better way of putting it.

A contributing factor to sickness is that we continue to eat the same kind of food as we age that we ate when we were younger.

Only one problem with this.

We cannot digest it properly now. And half-digested food finds its way into our colon!

It hasn't been digested so it sits there and it ROTS.

That is why when a person with this problem goes to the toilet the smell is like poison gas. The whole house stinks!

Yuk…

All that meat rotting away down there — no wonder there is such a smell. But there is something else happening…

Bad germs are proliferating. Billions and billions of them! Just like maggots around rotting meat in the sun. What a dreadful thought but that is how it is.

Did you know that six out of ten people who pass away die from 'diet induced disease'. This means that eating all the wrong things made it easy for the bad germs and viruses to overwhelm the body.

It means that the colon was unable to play its part in the defence of the body. It was too busy working overtime trying to do something about all that stuff being bunged down there every day. All that stuff lying there. All that stuff rotting away. All that stuff attracting all the wrong kind of bacteria. The bacteria that cause ill health not the bacteria essential for good health!

And this is happening in lots of people's colons every single day.

They are slowly dying from the colon up.

So the first step to build a bullet-proof colon is to look at what you eat. We talk about 'diets' as though this is some mysterious inner circle thing. A diet is simply the stuff we eat. That's it. Nothing else.

You can have a diet causing ill health.

You can have a diet causing good health.

And the choice is always yours. No-one else's. Just yours!

Choose right and you have an immune system that can beat the pants off anything. Choose wrong and you could find yourself in trouble.

Just like a modern city. Choose the right road and you end up in a leafy suburb, lovely homes, peaceful and law-abiding. Choose the wrong road and you end up in a slum where your very life is in danger.

There is not a lot to remember really. You don't need a book on diet. You don't need daily lectures. You just have to follow a few basic rules.

Remember, where there are rules there is order. Where there are no rules you have chaos.

Here are some simple tips to ensure you have a great colon, digestion and as a result a stronger immune system.

Remember, I said as we grow older we cannot digest the same as we used to. We need help. We don't like to admit that we can't do today what we did so easily some years ago. Or was it only yesterday? It doesn't seem all that long ago when we could eat whatever was put in front of us.

Poor digestion creeps up on us.

A common cause of trouble as we age is the fact we put out less hydrochloric acid in our stomachs. And what this means, my friend, is we find it harder and harder to digest protein.

Beans give us wind. And bad smelling wind at that! When we break wind, grown men writhe in agony, women faint and the dog runs out of the house! Well, probably not quite that bad, but bad enough.

Meat sits there. A lump of cement in the pit of our stomach. Slowly rotting away because of our lack of hydrochloric acid to digest it. And here is the bad news. A lot of bowel cancers are caused by this undigested protein sitting in our bowels.

And irritable bowels are everywhere. And every second person seems to be complaining about diverticulitis. And even more amazing, these complaints are not confined to one particular country.

They are international problems.

Which is comforting in a way. Shows we are all human and

subject to the same laws. Even more encouraging is that the help is also international. What helps one person over here also helps another person over there. There doesn't seem to be any special rules just applying to one lot of human beings and not to another.

So let us press on...

A good idea for colon health, health generally, is to cut down on meat. Lean meat, fat meat, in-between meat... all meat.

When I look at the average meal plate there is usually a heap of meat, a heap of potatoes and some vegetables.

At the end of the meal the meat has all gone. There may be a bit of token fat on the side of the plate. But most of it has gone!

The potatoes have all gone too. Down the hatch. Especially if they have been soaked in butter or cream. Mmmm, yummie! But deadly!

And if anything is left, it is the vegetables. Poor things.

Now come on, we all know deep down that this is wrong. At the beginning the servings could have been better arranged. Try this on for size. The largest portion on the plate should be the vegetables.

And not boiled. I have mentioned this earlier but it bears repeating. Do not boil your vegetables. It makes them soggy. It leaches out all the goodness. So steam them, wok them, eat them raw but don't boil them.

One potato is enough. We used to play a game when I was a kid called 'one potato, two potato' but this may well apply to a rhyme when using a skipping rope, but not to your meal plate. One small to medium sized potato is enough.

And the meat should be the smallest portion on your plate.

Huge T-Bones, New Yorkers, a hunk of meat so large it hangs over the sides of the plate, are a health hazard.

So I encourage you to eat a lot more vegetables. Eat lots of fruits. I eat apples, pears, soft fruits when in season. I eat lots of salads. I have a large salad every day for lunch. I do not eat meat at all. But that is my preference. I like a variety of vegetables.

Get variety into your meals.

And this means moving out of your meal 'comfort zone'.

My wife, Peg, will tell you I have no idea what is in our refrigerator. That is because it never occurs to me to eat between meals.

I do not spend my day raiding the fridge. And that is not because I am some sort of dietary saint. It is because I eat a hearty breakfast of unsweetened muesli with soy milk. This is slow digesting so I feel full. I am not attacked by hunger pains.

A large plate of salad with vegie pie or some fish is lunch. I always have chopped-up fruits as a dessert. And at night, more vegetables. Food I have grown to like are things like Peg's vegetable pie, where she uses baked rice instead of pastry. I love her vegetable lasagna… I am lucky. My dear wife is totally supportive in my battle against cancer. She comes up with delicious imaginative meals.

Whoever said vegetarian meals were dull has never eaten at our home!

I have conditioned myself not to eat salt. So we cook without salt.

It is always a source of wonder to me when we go out dining to see people sprinkling salt and pepper on their meal **before they have even tasted it**! I ask the waiter to tell the chef not to put salt on the meal he is preparing for me. It is my opinion there is too much salt on food you get in most restaurants already without putting more on.

I hasten to interject that some people do need salt. In fact, we all need salt. But not the bleached, chemically altered stuff we happily call salt. The only salt worth eating in my humble opinion is the natural salt. This comes usually as Celtic Salt. One of the best sources is Northern France. Look for it in your Health and Nutrition Centre. It is more expensive than the white stuff but it is good for you. The white stuff isn't!

Sesame seeds are great… they taste like salt. Try some, you will be amazed. Put some in soups and you will think salt has been added.

I don't eat sugar either. It is my belief that sugar is one of the inner enviromental curses of modern life. Kids get loaded with it. And we wonder why there are so many hyperactive children around these days.

The poor little mites are loaded up with sugar, artificial colourings, artificial preservatives and who knows what else. And we take them to the psychiatrist. Perhaps we are taking the wrong person.

Get sugar out of your diet as far as you can. It is very difficult because even so-called health bars are loaded with sugar.

Simple foods are best.

If you have cancer and want to take charge of your life, change your diet. If you don't want cancer, look carefully at your diet. And that simply means all the foods you shove in your mouth.

A WORD ABOUT ALCOHOL

You could say that alcohol is the lubricating oil of our modern society. The dumb become talkative. The timid brave. Marvellous are the effects of alcohol.

At least, that is what we are led to believe.

There are more illegitimate babies born these days than ever before. And this despite the 'worldliness' of modern teenage girls. But when alcohol is in, all restraint tends to go out… the guard goes down.

More murders are committed when people are overloaded with drink. More bashings. More domestic violence.

And for the guy with prostatic cancer the news is even worse.

And for the guy with an enlarged prostate…

The bad news is alcohol goes straight to your prostate. It HATES it! If you have too much alcohol, and for some people one glass of wine is too much, you find it difficult to empty your bladder.

You go to the pub or a restaurant. You are having a good time. The conversation is great. You don't notice how much wine is going down. That is until you go to the toilet.

And you stand there for what seems like forever waiting for the urine to flow. When it does come it doesn't actually *flow*. More like a drop by drop dribble. There you stand absolutely bursting. And next to nothing is leaking out.

Because your prostate has just enlarged and is choking off the flow from your bladder. So it is a good idea to listen to your body. And this means cutting out or very much down on alcohol.

Develop a winning personality without alcohol.

Your life could depend on it. High stakes, indeed.

OXYGENATING THE BOWEL

Did you realise you can go to the toilet every day and still be constipated? Yes, that's right. Go every day and be constipated. Doesn't sound right does it?

But it's true!

What happens is the lining of the bowel is encrusted with ancient rubbish, It has become hard, like concrete. It stops your bowel from contracting. It slows down the flow to a dead stop. The bowel is no longer urging the wastes along.

So you take laxatives. And these sell by the ton in our modern world. Billions of people feel they cannot go to the toilet without a laxative.

But all they pass is the central core. The bulk of the stuff sits there. Putrifying. Poisoning the system. Weakening your body. Making it hard to fight cancer or anything else. Clogging up your immune system.

So it is important to get rid of this accumulated waste.

There are a number of ways for you to do this. An obvious way is by reforming the diet. Eat bulk foods. Get fibre into your diet from plenty of fruits and vegetables. You can get ready-made preparations that are not laxatives, but which help to relieve the load on the colon. These usually have ingredients such as psyllium husks, slippery elm bark, oat bran, linseed and are flavoured with something natural like carob.

There is also another way gaining favour. This is to take small amounts of oxygen into the system. There are patented products on the market. But I suggest you go to a qualified Naturopath for advice on these products. The theory is that by increasing oxygen and magnesium in the bowel you can get rid of the accumulated wastes and end up with a vibrantly healthy colon.

Worth investigating. So many diseases are reputed to originate in the colon that a healthy colon is essential.

We all need a colon that works. Some people say it is fine to empty the bowel every three or four days. Nonsense! If the bowel is not emptying, it is filling. And filling with stuff that should be passed out every single day. Not every three or four days.

Drink plenty of fluid every day. And fluid does not mean coffee. Caffeine is bad for the prostate. It doesn't like it. It doesn't make much sense to drink something to make the prostate worse. That's the last thing we want. So cut out coffee and alcohol. It may be hard.

People cry to me 'But what else can I drink?'

As though coffee or tea are the only drinks out there.

I drink ginseng tea. I drink dandelion coffee. I drink the Ayerverdic teas for Vata, Pitta and Kapha to get my body in balance.

And I only drink water that has been purified. I never drink water out of a tap. I consider it a chemical menace. I urge you to drink plenty of water but only filtered water.

So to boost the immune system, one of the things you must do is to attend to the health of the bowel and digestive system.

Cut down on meat, coffee, sugar and sweet things. Eat lots

of fruits, vegetables, salads, wholemeal bread (never white), brown rice and wholesome foods.

Make sure you have plenty of fibre in your diet. If necessary, look for a preparation with Psyllium husks, linseed, slippery elm bark, oat bran and rice bran, using a natural flavouring such as carob.

Eat your way back to health. You will have a hard job beating your health problems if you do not change what you eat. Have you heard the old saying 'If you keep doing what you've always done, you'll get what you've always got!' And if you are like me, you don't like what you have got and want to do something about it.

So do what I did and still do — look after bowel health with good eating.

In the next chapter I will tell you more of the little known herbs I used to beat my so-called incurable cancer.

9 Let us turn the tables on cancer!

Cancer has had its own way for too long, in my opinion. It is time to turn the tables. Let us give cancer a hard time instead of the other way round.

I looked at ways to stop the testosterone turning into the DHS, the bad stuff and I looked at ways to starve the cancer cells of blood.

In military terms I intended to stop the enemy landing more troops and intended to cut the lines of supply. This is a very effective way of dealing with an enemy.

So how could I stop the blood supply to the cancer mass?

As I remarked earlier, cancer cells need a lot of extra blood. They are bigger than ordinary cells and reproduce at a faster rate. So they need lots of blood to do this.

And had to find ways to stop their blood supply. To strangle the horrible little monsters.

The first one I discovered was Red Clover, which I mentioned earlier. It's funny but I had known about certain healing qualities of this humble little plant.

I had used it for skin complaints for years. Trifolium (which means 'three leaves') has been used for skins for years. I also knew that lately it has been discovered to help women with menopausal problems such as hot flashes.

But then I found out that Red Clover is very helpful for the male reproductive system too. And even more important, found out that it contains Geniston.

And Geniston has the power to slow down the blood supply to cancers. And for me and you that was a momentous discovery.

I had said in an early chapter I thought the cancer research should concentrate more on ways to stop the testosterone converting to DHA and stopping the blood supply to the cancers.

And they were growing in my front lawn... the answer was sitting there all the time. Just that I was too uninformed to see.

So now I was excited!

If Red Clover had this ability, there must be other herbs with a similar ability.

What were they? How could I find them?

I mentioned earlier the herb Saw Palmetto. With your permission I would like to repeat what I said earlier about this herb.

My reason for taking Saw Palmetto is because it alleviates an enlarged prostate by inhibiting the conversion of testosterone into Dihydrotestosterone, the bad guy in this scenario.

It also speeds up the excretion of DHA out of the prostate gland. And this improves a lot things.

I believe that my problem was not too much testosterone. I repeat what I said before, I believe the problem is the conversion of whatever testosterone I had to the bad version, Dihydrotestosterone.

And Saw Palmetto was an important herb, an important alternative, something to keep testosterone safe!

As an interesting aside, I read that whilst orthodox medical opinion is all about stopping the production of testosterone, there is a growing body of opinion discrediting this point of view.

Would you believe that in one medical paper I read, the writer said: 'Testosterone is widely regarded by orthodox medical practitioners as "feeding" Prostate Cancer cells. This theory is now discredited and it is speculated that ***testosterone may even help to prevent Prostate Cancer!***' (the italics are mine).

Unfortunately, the writer didn't elaborate on this statement, so I don't know what was his basis for it. But it is interesting, isn't it?

THE AMAZING ACTION OF ZINC

For a long time I have told male patients of mine who are over 40 to take zinc. Why? Because zinc is essential for a male healthy reproductive system.

You know, when a childless couple is presented to the family doctor because the woman can't get pregnant, suspicion automatically falls on her. She is subjected to tests of all kinds. She it told to relax, don't make a business of what should be simply pleasure.

And the man stands there in his armour-plated opinion that it must be his partner's fault. It never occurs to him that he could play a part in the failure to conceive.

Ah, such is our male vanity and our male pride... 'Me? In some way responsible. Are you kidding?'

But quite often the problem lies with the male of the species. Sorry guys, but this is a fact. Tough, I know, but a fact just the same.

Now before you start climbing into the defensive armour just listen to this for a moment. Men with a low sperm count are most always low in zinc. Men with sperm that hates Monday mornings, that is slow off the mark, that finds swimming up the tube to the egg too much of an effort are usually low in zinc.

And quite often men with an enlarged prostate gland are low in zinc.

You don't produce zinc in your body

Too much copper depresses zinc levels. And where would a nice person like you get too much copper? Well, strange as it may seem, from the water pipes in your house if they are made from copper. Most modern water systems use copper piping and a tiny amount leaches into the water. It doesn't take much to do a job on you.

So copper can be a culprit.

The other one is diet. Zinc is found mainly in seafoods. That's one of the reasons people say oysters are an aphrodisiac... because they are rich in zinc. But how many oysters a day do you eat?

Another very good source of zinc is pumpkin seeds. Chomp on these all say long and you will get a fair whack of zinc.

Another problem we have is modern food processing. Food processing removes zinc from the food being processed. For example, 80% of the zinc is removed from flour in the processing. Zinc is water soluble and goes down the drain when vegetables are boiled. When you defrost frozen vegetables, the zinc disappears.

So as you can see, getting zinc from our diet is a problem.

And you'll never guess the major way we lose zinc from our bodies... SEX. Yes, good old sex. Every time you have sex, my friend, and ejaculate you lose 15mg of zinc each time. And this is the cruncher. We men need 15mg a day to stay healthy. So there is another important reason why we should take a zinc supplement.

According to Doctor Carl Pfeiffers most of the population are borderline deficient in zinc. No wonder we have so many prostate problems.

ZINC CAN DO A GOOD JOB IN RELIEF FROM PROSTATE CANCER

From my point of view, there is another powerful reason for taking extra zinc. And I urge you to make zinc as part of your daily routine to prevent prostate problems.

But I urge you to take it even more if you have prostate cancer.

And here is why... zinc inhibits the conversion of testosterone to very undesirable dihydrotestosterone. And we know that it is this that 'feeds' the cancer that is trying to kill us!

There is an old saying 'Physician Heal Thyself' and just as they say the shoemaker's shoes are always in need of repair so all too often health professionals whilst giving patients good advice do not always take it themselves.

And I have to tell you that was the case with me. I knew all about zinc being necessary for male health but I thought my diet was enough. It wasn't! And I paid the price.

Prostate Cancer!

So now I added zinc to my weapons for stopping testosterone being converted to Dihydrotestosterone.

THERE ARE OTHER REASON FOR TAKING ZINC

Zinc helps to reduce the size of an enlarged prostate and this can be a real blessing.

An enlarged prostate can cause infection of the bladder. An infected bladder can cause you unlimited trouble. Pain, difficulty in passing water, so much so they may have to put a tube (called a 'catheter') up your penis to relieve the pressure. Not a nice thought, but can be a life-saver.

If you cannot get rid of the urine in your bladder it will back up into the kidneys. And then you have a real problem on your hands. You will have to get into hospital pretty damn quick. If you don't you could die of Uric Acid poisoning.

An enlarged prostate can obstruct the neck of the bladder and make you wet your pants. This is embarrassing. Who wants to find he can't make it to the toilet and have a large wet stain at the front of his pants? Not you or me, eh?

If you have an enlarged prostate then you already know it can get you out of bed umpteen times a night. You wake up tired out. Your partner is kept awake by your nightly trips, and she doesn't like it. So you have two tired and grumpy people. Not the best of situations!

These are all good reasons for you to take zinc even if you don't have cancer.

By the way, you may be reading this book because you don't want a problem. It may be that you are fine at the moment but are sensibly finding out the options. Well, you too would benefit from taking zinc.

Because zinc should be part of every man's prostate hygiene regime.

So take zinc to inhibit the conversion of testosterone to dihydrotestosterone if you are in the position I was in, that is if you have prostate cancer. Do take it to help reduce the size of your prostate if you are suffering from an enlarged prostate. And take it to make sure you don't have either of these problems further along your Life journey.

Most instructions about taking zinc
are wrong

You may be surprised to learn that most of the time the directions on the bottle of zinc you have bought are wrong. Yes, that's what I said, most times the directions are wrong.

On the bottle it usually tells you to take one tablet three times a day with meals. Right? Wrong, wrong, wrong!

Zinc binds with certain elements in food. So when you take it with food more often than not it is not available to your body. In other words, you did your dough! You conscientiously take your zinc three times a day thinking it is doing you good.

And it isn't! Because it is not there for your body to absorb. It has been blocked by elements in the meal you just ate.

So the best time, the only time, to take zinc is either last thing at night or first thing in the morning. Ignore the directions on the bottle if it says take it with meals. Listen to me, take it either first thing in the morning or last thing at night.

I take mine last thing at night because that is the most convenient time for me.

More to tomatoes than meets the eye

Hey, did you know that tomatoes were once called 'love apples'?

Now that is very interesting. Why? Because the prostate gland is very much involved in love. In fact, one of the first signs the prostate is failing is when attempts at love-making fail.

And the love apple, the tomato, is it another everyday vegetable or is it a fruit? Anyway, whatever it is, the tomato can help you reduce an overgrown prostate.

This is because tomatoes have a substance in them called Lycopene. It's funny how things turn out. To get Lycopene you have to cook the tomato. Your body can't get the Lycopene from raw tomatoes, they have to be cooked or a paste.

Lycopene is what they call a 'carotene'. This is the stuff you get from carrots. And the one from carrots is called Beta-Carotene. And Beta-Carotene is one powerful anti-oxidant. You will remember I told you earlier that oxidants (free radicals is another term) are the evil little blighters that cause all the damage to our bodies.

So an anti-oxidant is something that knocks the little monsters on the head. Gobbles them up. Gives them the old 'one two' as the old-time boxers used to say.

And Lycopene is also a heavy-hitter when it comes to anti-oxidant activity. In fact, this meek ingredient of the tomato is the heaviest hitter out of 500 different anti-oxidants. If I were a Free Radical busily causing prostate cancer and I had the chance of seeing Lycopene bearing down on me I would run for cover as fast as I could.

But Lycopene could outrun me.

Researchers have pointed to the fact that Italian men are less likely to get prostate cancer than other men and postulate that this may be because they eat tomatoes with almost everything.

Lycopene to be effective must be eaten with dietary oil. And look at the Italians. What do they eat? Loads of tomato paste together with olive oil. So without realising it, they are eating a great anti-prostate cancer diet.

You can now get Lycopene in tablets or capsules from any decent Health and Nutrition Centre. And the only side effect is that you will get a sun tan without going out in the sun. Wow, now what drug could do that for you?

More help against cancer from the garden

Have you ever thought what a wonderful world we live in?

I have said this before but it bears repeating. It amazes me how there are flowers, herbs, weeds (!), minerals, vegetables — all sorts of natural plants that we take for granted.

And yet so many of them have a secret locked away inside of them. They have something or other that is **specific** for some human complaint. I find this marvellous. It strongly confirms my belief in a Cosmic Mind. I find it impossible to believe that all these wonders came about by accident. Just by chance, Saw Palmetto is a terrific anti-cancer agent specifically for the prostate gland. Just by chance, Epilobium, the small willow herb, is a **specific** for reducing an enlarged prostate.

Just by chance? They've got to be kidding!

And there is another vegetable in your garden that is a potent anti-cancer agent. It sits there all innocent looking. No-one would believe the hidden power in it. People eat it every day in salads.

It is the common beetroot.

I love beetroots. Peg cooks a whole pan full for me and I eat the lot. I have beetroot grated raw on salads. Delicious! Very crunchy... Mmmm!

I think that my love of beetroots has helped me win the battle against cancer. I really do think that.

Let me tell you more about the beetroot.

Did you know that the beetroot is one of the best liver herbs you can get? I recommend raw beetroot juice as part of a detox programme. This is because it is so effective in helping the liver.

Do you know where your liver is in your body? It is roughly under the bottom of your right rib cage. If your liver is a bit off and you push up under the right rib you will usually feel a bit sick. Nausea rears its ugly head.

Beetroot is best eaten raw as an anti-cancer, liver boosting agent. Unlike tomatoes which are best cooked.

So add raw beetroots to your list of anti-cancer agents. Gradually you are building up a fearsome armoury against cancer.

Now I know I repeat myself so don't write and tell me. I know. And I repeat myself for a purpose. Like any good friend I sincerely want to help you get better.

And being human we forget things. We don't take any notice when people talk to us. We are not always paying attention.

Remember how many times your Mum had to shout to get you to hear? Even something important like tea-time. 'This is the last time I'll call you. You come here **right now**!' And finally we would realise that Mum was actually shouting at us.

Well, it's the same with me. I like to repeat things so it gets into your psyche. I want it to become part of your every day thinking.

So when you see beetroots you will automatically say to your partner: 'Oh, great, beetroots today. Good, oh, by the way, don't boil them. I love them RAW. Grate them up and put a pile on my salad. Oh yes, and let's have a pasta, with lots of good old tomato paste on it'.

Now who in the world would realise that you were beating the heck out of prostate cancer? I tell you, my friend, it really is a wonderful world.

WHY YOU SHOULD EAT RICE AND NOT POTATOES

Brown rice is a food that is also recommended as an anti-prostate cancer food. We normally pile up our plate with potatoes. I guess that potatoes are the most eaten vegetable ever. We have them boiled, we have them fried, we have them done in their jackets, we have them as so-called 'french fries'. We slice them, we grate them, we eat them whole, we put them in soups, we use potato flour. It is quite amazing the ways in which we use potatoes. They are part of our way of life.

But I want to suggest to you something unthinkable. Eat less potatoes and eat more brown rice.

Because rice reduces the incident of prostate cancer.

And because a major predisposing factor to prostate cancer is FAT and all too often we eat potatoes fried or covered in butter or cream, they do not help our cause at all.

If you eat a potato, and I love them, eat them done in their jacket without the cream or butter. Oh I know it's a bit of a thing when a fellow can't enjoy a blooming potato drenched in cream or lashing of butter. It's a cruel world. And doing without potatoes and fatty dressings is a small price to pay to enjoy the magic of this so-called 'cruel world' for many more years to come.

And that is my sincerest wish for you. That is why I sat for hours on end writing this book. Because I want you to enjoy life for many more productive years.

Can I make this point? There is a bond between us. We both want to drive away the grim spectre of death by prostate cancer. I have done it, and I know you can too. We are friends, you and I. We have this single goal.

We don't want prostate cancer, we don't want an enlarged prostate and sure as hell we don't want to die of prostate cancer.

So, friend, we do what we have to do. Right? Of course!

So moving on together...

Let me say to you while the thought is in my head (I told you this book is more like a conversation between two mates than a lecture on prostate or other cancers). If you are already on chemo, listen up.

One of the problems of chemotherapy and radiation is losing your hair, feeling sick as a dog and often finding out it wasn't all that crash hot a remedy after all.

To dramatically minimise the side effects of chemo/radiation assault, take loads of Vitamin C like I told you before. But also take the amino acid Glutamine.

Glutamine helps to minimise the damage caused by radiation. It also helps to repair the damage to the intestines caused by radiation.

And here is something quite remarkable (I told you it's a magic world we live in). When Glutamine is given along with chemotherapy, tumours decrease in size by up to 45%. Now if that isn't a miracle, what the heck is? And folks on chemo stand a much better chance of survival if they take Glutamine along with the chemo.

Glutamine will relieve the pain of the sores in the mouth caused by chemotherapy. And if that weren't enough, Glutamine stimulates the growth of Lymphocytes and also the growth of Phagocytes. These are the warrior class, the Samurai of the cells. They are the boys you want on your side in spades.

Now you may be asking yourself: If Glutamine is so brilliant, why don't doctors use it as part of their medical procedures when dosing people up with chemo and radiation?

And the answer is blindingly simple, good friend.

It is because they don't know about it.

Now let's be fair to your hard working family doctor. By

and large they have a hard life. Doctors die younger than the rest of us. Seeing loads of patients every day. Expected to be like God. At the risk of being sued for everything they have if they make an un-God-like decision that causes someone a problem. Never mind the thousands of good decisions they make, just make one mistake and you could be a goner. I would not like to be a doctor myself, would you?

Members of my family are doctors and I love them dearly. And I would not like their workload one little bit. So when I say things about the medical profession I am not knocking doctors. I might be knocking the attitudes they absorb at Medical School where I believe they teach a lot of old fashioned out-of-date attitudes. But I admire doctors.

But that doesn't alter the fact that they can't know everything about everything. And they don't. And it is the same when it comes to prostate cancer.

They are usually well-informed about the standard medical procedures. Drugs, Chemo, Radiation and Surgery. Because that is part of their everyday life. They have the sad task of sending patients to Urologists, Cancer specialists... then the even worse task of reading you the letter they got from the specialist.

Like the one my doctor read to me.

So it is not surprising they do not know about Glutamine or any of the other treatments we are discussing together. In fact, do your doctor a favour and give him a copy of this book. Hopefully, it will open his or her eyes.

Expecting a doctor to know all about alternative ways to treat cancer is like expecting your local family butcher to be a vegetarian!

So let us press on.

Add Glutamine to your impressive list of weapons to beat cancer. You can get Glutamine without prescription at any Health and Nutrition Centre. And it has no side effects.

Here is a couple of bonus tips about Glutamine if you have

any doubts at all about taking it. Glutamine is essential for healthy DNA. And it is maverick DNA that is causing the problem. Hey, and if you are miserable about cutting down on alcohol as part of your winning campaign against cancer, Glutamine helps to reduce the craving for alcohol. And if you are a trifle overweight, it also reduces the craving for sugar.

Now isn't that terrific? So get into it!

You want more? More about Glutamine?

OK, we're friends, so here goes...

Glutamine alleviates male impotence. That short sentence carries a load of meaning. Yes, Glutamine helps to stiffen the vital organ and can transform an otherwise dull life.

It can help to reduce tiredness. And let's face it. One of the most common excuses and reasons for a poor sex life is 'I'm too tired tonight'.

Glutamine helps with Alzheimers Disease. Surely one of the fastest growing problems in our society today. A major problem facing doctors is that patients forget they have taken their pills and take them again and again! So anything that helps this destruction of our memory is welcome. Write it down before you forget! (That was hopefully a joke.)

Glutamine reduces aggressive behaviour. Not just because it reduces the amount of alcohol people pour into themselves. It acts on the brain. Because of its action in the brain it also helps concentration.

In fact, is does a lot of things to help the areas of our lives where we tend to need a lot of help.

And for people who are unhappily going for surgery, Glutamine is one of the most important nutrients to give people before and after surgery.

Definitely one of Nature's wonders.

THIS IS A HERB YOU MUST HAVE...

Put the herb Astragalus at the top of your list of herbs that will help you back into a vital and vibrant cancer-free life.

And Astragalus is an important herb for anyone who wants to do something sensible to protect himself against cancer of any kind. Ask any Herbalist, they will tell you what a mighty herb we have in Astragalus.

Astragalus is one big buddy when it comes to the immune system. Now you remember all I have told you about your immune system. Remember I said if anyone had cancer the first thing to do is to strengthen the host. That is make your body battleship-proof against attack by viruses, bacteria or robber gangs of cells.

And this is where Astragalus is like steel reinforcing concrete. It is a deep immune system restorative. It really get the immune system going. Which is just what we want, isn't it?

We need to get our big guns out and all firing… Boom, Boom. BOOM!!! And that is precisely what Astragalus does.

It is known as a 'deep immune system' booster.

Have you heard of Echinacea? This a fabulous herb. It is another immune system booster. But it does not goes as deep as Astragalus. It is fine for protecting oneself against going down with influenza. It is great for helping a person to get over influenza. And taken with Vitamin C it is a cheap insurance against winter colds and sickness.

But Astragalus is more powerful. If Echinacea is the Armoured Personnel Carrier, Astragalus is the mighty, heavily armoured tank. It lumbers into battle formidably armed and creating havoc among the enemy.

Just what we want!

So let you and me find out some more about this herb…

Research has shown that Astragalus DOUBLES survival time of cancer patients. This of itself is pretty strong stuff. I doubt if Chemo or Radiation doubles survival time. And look at the price the patient has to pay for having Chemo or Radiation. Very high! And unpleasant. And nasty!

So something that helps without side effects is welcome, right?

Astragalus originally came from Northern China and was, and is, a basic part of Chinese Medicine. Did you know that the oldest text book on medicine is Chinese? It was commissioned something like 5,000 years ago by the 'Yellow Emperor'. That is what they called him. And that book is still around in China and still being used.

When your body attacks cancer it does it with what are called Interferons. Interferons were popular medicine some time ago. The pharmaceutical companies produces a drug called Interferon to stimulate the production of interferon in the fight against cancer.

Well, Astragalus does this naturally.

But like so many herbs, there are wonderful side effects.

And Astragalus is no exception!

It helps digestion. And as any Naturopath will tell you, helping the digestion is a major plank in devising ways to help patients back to health.

It speeds up the Basal Metabolic Rate. Now who do you think would just love to have that piece of information? Anyone who is carrying too much weight. That's who. Because speeding up the metabolic rate speeds up the rate of burn. People with a high metabolic rate do not usually put weight on. This is good stuff!

Do you remember how I told you about your adrenal glands? OK, so you forgot. Well, that's a pretty human thing to do. Anyway I'll refresh your memory.

Your adrenal glands sit over your kidneys and are major energy glands. The stresses of modern life tend to deplete the supply of adrenaline. Even worse, they slow down the adrenal glands' ability to produce it. And you need adrenaline for energy. You need it for excitement. You need it for enthusiasm.

You gotta have adrenaline. You don't want too much, of course, but you want enough. And a lot of people do not have enough.

On a world trip Peg and I made some years ago, we came to

the conclusion that tiredness was an international condition. How did we arrive at this conclusion? Because whenever anyone found out I am a Naturopath they asked for help with tiredness. And this was true wherever we went.

A sure price we are paying for so-called progress. The word progress means movement. And progress can mean movement forward or backward. I sometimes wonder about progress in the modern world, don't you?

Anyway, philosophy aside, Astragalus helps tiredness because it is a tonic for the adrenal glands. It is also great for improving stamina — they found that mice supplemented with Astragalus could swim for longer than mice without it.

The Chinese say Astragalus is very beneficial for strengthening the lungs in cases of lung weakness.

So all in all, I take Astragalus every day as part of my anti-cancer regime and I recommend it to you.

That is enough for today. It is a good idea to keep reading and re-reading each chapter. You will find each time you read the same chapter again you will get something else from it.

It takes repetition for our minds to accept things. And a lot of what I am telling you will be very new to you. It is not part of accepted wisdom about fixing cancer. We also have to contend with conditioning.

By that I mean we have been conditioned since birth to believe that drug medicine is the only way to go. It is bred into us. In some ways suggesting that medicine does not have all the answers is like attacking motherhood.

I used to live in a country area that relied heavily on dairy. Lots of dairy herds around. And there was I telling people that dairy was probably bad for them. I think a lot of people who go around complaining of sinus really have a milk allergy. If they stopped drinking milk, things would improve. Dairy products make mucus in a lot of people. Dairy is not the best for people with cancer, in my opinion.

When I suggest to people that they give up dairy they cried:

'But what about my bones? What about my calcium?' I can only reply by asking where does the elephant get its calcium. It has stronger bones than you and I.

I would suggest you do as I do. Get your calcium from Soy products. Tofu. Tempeh, Miso and Soy Milk. On the point of Soy Milk, be aware that chemical companies are breeding hybrid soy plants that can withstand enormous amounts of pesticides. And despite the protestations to the contrary, I believe that residual pesticides get into these soy beans.

If you need convincing, listen to this bit of information. Agitation is going on to make the chemical companies declare on the packet that the soy used in the product is from chemically drenched plants.

And the chemical companies are resisting this with all their might and money! I wonder why? Why don't they want you to know?

Because they know you are not stupid. They know you would not buy the product. And this would harm profits. And believe it or not, these people are far more concerned with profit than they are with your good health.

In the olden days I reckon I would have been burned at the stake for heresy. In modern times they burn you at the stake by attacking your reputation. Have you noticed how politicians and spokespeople for various professional bodies express their opinions as though they were FACTS. And what are they really? Opinions, that's all. Opinions!

Politicians, columnists and other people who fancy themselves as formers of public opinion will state something as a fact. Hitler was a master at this caper. He made what were and are ridiculous statements about the Jewish people as though they were facts. And people in Germany accepted these dangerous opinions as facts. And look at the savagery that provoked.

Have you noticed how newspapers these days make outrageous statements about people in the public eye as though they are announcing some recently discovered 'fact'. These again are opinions.

And remember this, a medical diagnosis is an opinion and not necessarily a fact.

So when you are reading this book, try to get out of your mind most of what you have been led to believe. Drugs are not the only way. Chemicals, Radiation, Surgery are not your only options.

But I tell you about opinions being taken as facts because it is hard for us to go against our conditioning. It takes courage.

So read and re-read each chapter. Take notes. Write down what you have read in your own words. Marvellous for remembering what you have read. Underline important sentences. This way when you go back to your book you can 'skim' and get all the information that is important to you.

OK, my friend, so let us now go ahead. In the next chapter I am going to introduce you to something very exciting in the battle against cancer. I believe this stuff is a major factor in my spectacular release from the death row of cancer victims.

So listen to what I have to say. What you read will probably surprise you but it will help you too, believe me!

10 This could be the 'Atomic Bomb' of cancer remedies!

Do you remember when I was talking about positive selective perception? This is when you suddenly see things of interest to you in fulfilling your breakthrough goal.

You suddenly notice articles that you had never seen before. In my case, being a Naturopath, I noticed all the articles on prostate cancer in the journals, newsletters and monographs I receive.

I also noticed that I met more men with prostate problems than ever before. I believe I attracted these people because that's where my focus was.

And remarkably, with positive selective perception you seem to attract to yourself not only people, articles and so on, but other things.

And so it was with me!

I am inclined to be somewhat untidy. I never throw papers away. I accumulate them. I have piles of magazines on health, articles, books, papers, notes and heaven knows what else around all the time.

One day, going through one of the piles I noticed a small book. Only 24 pages. It was by a Doctor John F. Prudden and I had no idea where it had come from.

Obviously, when I got it, from wherever that was, I wasn't interested. I hadn't read it. I had just added it to the pile.

But this particular day, for no apparent reason, I decided to go through this pile. And found the book.

As I said, it was only 24 pages. But I remembered what one of my teachers had told me years ago: 'Anyone who thinks you buy information by the pound is a fool'. One page of information could be worth ten thousand dollars.

'Oh, hold on!' you might think 'Ten thousand dollars for one page, that's asking a bit much'.

OK, but let me ask you a question.

If I could give you information, on one page, that guaranteed you income for life, what would it be worth? Not a catch. Genuine, tested information that guaranteed you financial security for the rest of your life.

What would you pay for it? Especially if it came with a money-back guarantee? Five thousand dollars? Ten thousand dollars?

Such a piece of paper would be worth a fortune but it is only one page!

There is no such piece of paper that I am aware of. Sorry to build up your hopes… but you can see what I am driving at.

It was the same with this little 24-page booklet.. It astounded me.

I read it from cover to cover. I lapped it up. It seemed to speak directly to me. It hit the spot!

But I couldn't for the life of me remember where it came from. And without that knowledge I couldn't find out where to get the stuff Doctor Prudden was writing about.

EVEN MY HERBALIST FRIENDS DIDN'T KNOW

I phoned all the likely suppliers and they had never heard of the book nor the product Doctor Prudden was reporting on.

So I started phoning different herbalists I know. None seemed to know much about it.

After a lot of ringing around, I finally found a herbalist who said she had in fact heard of it. She told me to ring another herbalist who knew all about it, she was sure.

So I rang him... he had no idea but he told me to ring someone else who he was sure would know.

And this guy DID know. He told me who to ring and I finally tracked down the Australian manufacturer and his agent.

And guess what, the agent had been a friend of mine for over ten years. He was the one who had left the booklet with me and I had forgotten all about it..

But when I needed that information to save my life it miraculously appeared.

And now I shall share that information with you.

The book specifically dealt with
treating cancer

The booklet is all about treating cancer. Any kind of cancer.

Now I believe a lot of the information in this book you have in your hands is of great value to anyone suffering from cancer no matter where it is. And the discussion we are about to have is no exception.

The whole discussion in this book I found, is about what is called 'Bovine Tracheal Cartilage' and its use in treating different kinds of cancer, including prostate cancer.

It is interesting to note that Bovine Cartilage was first discovered to have therapeutic qualities as long ago as 1954. It was proven then that it helped amazingly with wound healing.

It was also shown to help spectacularly in a variety of complaints. These ranged from inflammatory conditions to cancer.

And yet it remains a mystery to most people. It must be one of the least known therapeutic agents in treating cancer. Even though it has a record that can only be described as fantastic.

Fasten your mental seat belt. This will be a rocky ride for anybody's long-held and cherished beliefs about cancer.

In the early days of research into the effectiveness of Bovine Tracheal Cartilage, 1,000 patients were involved. And a hundred of these were cancer patients!

What is more, after the initial treatment they were all followed-up and the results carefully written down... all very thorough.

Have you heard of something called 'serendipity'? This is when you happen upon something pleasant when doing something else. It is an unexpected happy result that just pops into person's life... just like that.

Doctor John Prudden was investigating the effectiveness of Bovine Cartilage by inserting little chips of it into cortisone-loaded rats. He had noticed the bad side effects of giving people cortisone and was looking for an effective alternative.

And he was experimenting with Bovine Cartilage as an alternative to the cortisone. He noticed something very interesting... the wounds treated with Bovine Cartilage healed up far more quickly. It reduced inflammation around the wound too. A double bonus, if you like.

This prompted John Prudden to make the study of Bovine Cartilage his life work.

And his discoveries will prove of great interest and importance to you as they were to me!

Doctor Prudden's breakthrough research turned out to be the foundation for all cartilage research. And this includes Shark Cartilage.

WHAT HAS SHINGLES GOT TO DO WITH CANCER?

I tell you what, one of the most painful of everyday illnesses is shingles. It is not so much the shingles itself but its aftermath. A lot of people have shingles neuralgia for years after the skin lesions have gone.

They say shingles is a sort of grown-up version of Chicken

Pox. But for the adult with it, shingles is ten times worse.

Shingles is called 'Herpes Zoster' and that should alert you to something. Yes, shingles belongs to the same family as cold sores, otherwise known as Herpes Simplex. And also to genital herpes. Not a nice family to know at all.

Now here is something interesting. When they exposed the herpes virus to Bovine Cartilage in test tubes, nothing happened. Yet in the body there were definite, measurable results.

The inevitable conclusion was that it was not the Bovine Cartilage itself that acted on the virus. No! It was the action of the Bovine Cartilage stimulating the immune system.

Once they realised this, intensive research began to find out how Bovine Cartilage performed its wonderful work.

You will remember how I suggested that cancer research would be well advised to spend time and money on stopping the cancer building up its blood supply. In the 1960s Doctor Judah Folkman, M.D. while working at the Harvard Medical School discovered something earthshaking in its importance to cancer patients.

Like many other doctors he knew that cancers need a lot more blood and he knew what they called 'angio-genesis' takes place where there is a cancer mass. This is a build up of a network of blood vessels especially to feed the tumour.

So his research centred on how to stop this network of blood vessels from building up. He needed proof that it was possible to stop this build up, a process called 'anti-angiogenesis'.

He saw this as an absolutely critical research. For if these blood vessels could be stopped from forming, if they could be choked off, then the cancer would die. It would die and wouldn't that be just fantastic!

A few years later, Robert Langer, D.Sc. and Anne Lee, Ph.D. of the Massachusetts Institute of Technology reported that Bovine Cartilage could inhibit the growth of blood vessel networks to solid tumours.

Other scientists reported that Bovine Cartilage is a biological response modifier that activates the ability of macrophages to destroy bacteria and viruses.

This simply means that Bovine Cartilage stimulates our own body to get in there and beat the hell out of cancer blood vessel networks. To knock bacteria and viruses silly.

This is the kind of stuff to get someone like me on the edge of my seat with excitement. Hope, real hope flooded me... my whole spirit lifted.

At that moment I just **KNEW** I was going to beat my prostate cancer! It was at that moment I gave myself six months to get it all under control.

EVEN AS A NATUROPATH I HAD NEVER HEARD OF BOVINE CARTILAGE!

Isn't it remarkable that even though I am a fully accredited Naturopath with over 15 years experience, I had never heard of Bovine Cartilage. I had heard of Shark Cartilage, especially since there had been a lot of publicity after a paper was read about it at a cancer convention in Canada. But nothing about Bovine Cartilage.

In fact, had I not found that little white booklet I probably still wouldn't have heard about it.

And that is why I am delighted to tell you about it.

Here is another brilliant option very few people need to know about. I have not met one patient with cancer who has heard of it. It certainly is not common knowledge among cancer specialists.

So all the more reason why you should know about it!

And that is why I am talking to you right now. You have a right to know ALL the options out there. This is knowledge that can save your life.

SEVEN MILLION DOLLARS OF RESEARCH...

Isn't it remarkable that over seven milllion dollars have been spent on research and so few people have heard of Bovine Cartilage.

Doctor Prudden's original research was all to do with wound healing. In fact, Bovine Cartilage is cited in medical text books in connection with its wound healing ability.

But it has more than that. A lot more as we will find out.

Doctor Prudden used Bovine Cartilage to treat a wide range of conditions... get this lot.

Cancer... yes, cancer. Including prostate cancer, breast cancer, cancer of the pancreas, brain, thyroid and squamous cancer of the nose and pharynx. An impressive list without any shadow of a doubt.

And I had never even heard of it!

But he used it for arthritis, allergies, skin diseases like Psoriasis and of course, herpes infections.

An awesome list, isn't it?

And waiting there for me to discover and now here for you! Which is great news.

How Bovine Cartilage affects the
Immune System

In our conversation together I keep harping on about the immune system. This is because I believe the Cosmic Intelligence didn't give us a partial immune system. We weren't given an immune system that works part time.

I believe we have a full on, hard hitting, ballistic immune system.

In the original Cosmic Plan we humans were intended to live for around 120 years. But we made a mess of it. We did everything wrong.

In the name of progress we have subjected our body to all sorts of things it was never intended to combat.

Just imagine the difference from the early days of the world. Impenetrable forests pouring oxygen into the air. Pure crystal clear rivers running down to a sea teeming with life. Humans running, gathering, bending, twisting... using their bodies every day. Because of their lifestyle breathing in deeply the crystal clear air... eating food straight from the vine, out of the rich black soil.

Contrast that with our lives today!

All the forests have gone. No longer pouring out life-giving oxygen. Nor mopping up carbon dioxide that is now creating the 'green house effect'. All in the name of progress.

The land has been stripped of its goodness. We have to continually overwhelm it with chemicals to grow anything at all. And they have what they call 'mono-crops'. Instead of a farm sowing many different crops in the fields, with one lying fallow, they now have vast tracts of land with only one crop. And this means they have to drench it with thousands of tons of chemicals to kill the bugs that now have no natural enemies.

This was not part of the original plan.

So now our immune system cannot cope. It has so much to contend with. Our poor liver is bashed about by all these chemicals it now has to try to get rid of. No wonder so many people are tired, sick and wonder what has gone wrong.

So where at one time our body would have dealt cancer a death dealing blow in one swoop, the cancer now deals us the death dealing blow. All because we have worked our immune system to exhaustion.

Compounding the problem is the love of antibiotics. As I remarked earlier, taking antibiotics not only knocks out the good guys that protect us they also make our immune system lazy.

You have heard the old saying 'If you don't use it... you lose it!'

This is just as true about our immune system. If we don't let it do its job properly, it stops doing it. And then we need more and more antibiotics for even the most trivial of problems.

And right now is where Bovine Cartilage comes galloping up like a knight in shining armour, pennants flying eager to help.

BOVINE DIDN'T WORK ON THE CANCER CELLS!

When the scientists tried out Bovine Cartilage on cancer cells in a Petrie Dish, nothing happened! And yet, in the body it worked!

So what was happening?

The only conclusion the scientists could come to was this. The Bovine Cartilage actually stimulated the immune system. And stimulated it to such an extent that it choked off the cancer cells.

More research uncovered something else quite strange. Bovine Cartilage stimulated the immune system to stop the cancer cells reproducing themselves. A very important and life-saving activity.

But Bovine Cartilage also worked on Rheumatoid Arthritis which is the immune system **attacking itself**! So now we had the puzzle, how could the Bovine do two things, stimulate the immune system and suppress it too?

Listen to what Doctor Prudden has to say about this: 'Bovine Cartilage is a "normaliser". Bovine Cartilage closely resembles what is called "fetal mesenchyme". This is the primordial tissue, the very stuff everything else is made from, the basic building material of the body. Fetal mesenchyme is the principal tissue from which muscle, bone, tendons, ligaments, skin, fat and bone marrow, which is the heart of the immune system, are made from.' And Bovine closely resembles this.

Isn't that a brain stopper of an idea? Incredible.

And great news for me and for you if you too have prostate cancer or are threatened with it!

This cartilage contains numerous powerful molecular biodirectors. These biodirectors have a powerful normalising effect on the multiple chemical and structural abnormalities of cancer cells!

I have written this statement of fact in bold type on purpose.

Read it again! Get the depth of this statement into your very tissues. What it is saying is here we have something that can **change** the way cancer cells operate. It can NORMALISE CANCER CELLS!

That statement had me almost crying with excitement.

I felt like a gold miner who had just struck the mother lode!

And incredibly, there is more! This is all exciting information!!

Doctor Brian Durie at the Department of Medicine, University of Arizona showed that Bovine had direct impact on cancer tissue. This revealed that Bovine not only stimulated the immune system but also attacked the cancer cells directly.

This was getting better and better!

He demonstrated that Bovine had a direct anti-mitotic effect on cancer cells. What that means in plain English, my friend, it that Bovine Cartilage stopped the cancer cells from dividing. It slows down the rate at which cancer cells replicate. Cancer cells normally 'clone' themselves rapidly. That is why cancer masses grow so dramatically in the body.

And Bovine Cartilage slowed this reproduction.

And the end result of this is death of the cancer!

How this happens they don't know. But it does!

They speculate that the Boving Cartilage's basic mucopolysaccharides act on the membrane of the cancer cells, stopping them from dividing.

Bovine gets the attacker cells into action

Doctor Prudden and his Associates discovered something else. Bovine Cartilage gets the macrophages, these devour foreign cells, into action. It not only does this, it also boosts the T cells and the B cells.

And this is fantastic news for anyone with cancer!

The B cells produce what are called immunoglobins A, G and M. And what these do, my friend, is increase the overall anti-mitotic activity. They stop the cancer cells from dividing and devouring healthy tissue. And often you will see an increase in natural killer cells!

I told you earlier that cancer cells are larger than normal cells and they can be measured. This is done with the ultimate power of the electron microscope which revealed that because of the magnificent way in which Bovine Cartilage stimulates the immune system, the malignant cells gradually decrease in size.

Now that's got to be the best news you have heard today!

THE DIFFERENCE BETWEEN BOVINE AND CHEMICAL WARFARE

Orthodox medicine uses chemicals and death rays to kill cancer cells. And this therapy can sometimes produce dramatic results but at great expense to the patient's immune system.

The patient's immune system is now less able to help itself.

Because of the limited success of chemicals and radiation, the pharmaccutical industry's attention have been drawn to immunotherapy.

However, **chemical** stimulation of the immune system has been notably unsuccessful. Agents like Interferon, Interleukins and Tumor Necrosis Factor, TNF, have been identified and isolated.

However, when large amounts of any of these agents are introduced into the immune system, the critical balance of the immune system is disrupted.

The results have been generally ineffective and toxic to the point of fatalities!

Not the best, eh?

Just listen to what Ralph Moss, Ph.D., author of *Cancer Therapy: The Independent Consumer's Guide* and *The Cancer Industry* had to say about these toxic substances. By the way, Ralph Moss is an expert on non-toxic cancer treatments. He is a member of the Board of Directors of the Office of Alternative Medicine at the National Institute of Health in America.

Remember, this man's whole life is dedicated to non-toxic

ways to help people with cancer and this is what he said about the pharmaceutical industry's efforts to chemically stimulate the immune system: 'Using these stimulants is like replacing the violin section with twice the number of trumpets in a finely-tuned philharmonic orchestra'.

Put simply, it is unbalanced overkill. Funny how we never hear about this kind of information.

Doctor Prudden's comments were that Bovine Cartilage selectively stimulates the immune system and normalises aberrant cells.

COULD BOVINE HELP PATIENTS WHERE STANDARD TREATMENT HAD FAILED?

Now let me tell you, this next bit is really interesting. Doctor Prudden decided to do a trial of Bovine Cartilage. Yes, but not your ordinary trial! No, he only accepted patients who 'Failed to respond to all standard therapy. Or people who had a cancer for which current therapy is generally recognised as ineffective'.

These are people who had abandoned hope. These were people whom the medical profession had written off. They would have been advised to take what is grimly called the 'Capri Option'. In plain English that means go home, get your affairs in order and try to have a good time in the short time you have left!

I find it hard to believe that anyone who had been given only a few months to live, someone who had been told 'there is nothing more we can do for you', would go home and enjoy themselves.

Doctor Prudden proved something very important. And if I have said this to you before, well, it deserves repeating. When a doctor or specialist says to you 'There is nothing more that can be done for you' he is talking medically.

What he is saying is true! But only if you think there is only one way to go. You see, when your specialist utters these fateful words he is speaking **medically**. Sure, there is no more drugs can do for you. There is no help coming from surgery. You can forget about radiation, you can forget about chemotherapy. They have all done their dash.

But he is wrong when he says there is nothing more that can be done.

In one breath he has wiped Herbal Medicine. He knows nothing about the wonderful things done with Homeopathy. He is unaware of the incredible results from mega-vitamin and other nutritional therapies. He has never believed in imaging for health... in short, he has wiped out a lot of therapies each of which has helped people with cancer.

And to me, even worse, the medical profession does not spend much effort on warning men over 40 of the dangers of an enlarged prostate and how this can lead to prostate cancer. The biggest cancer killer of men over 40 in our society today!

There is a lot of money being spent to warn women of the perils of breast cancer. They are urged repeatedly to get tested. Free testing! Get to it girls!

But as far as I can ascertain, not one zac telling the men to get tested for prostate problems. Yeah, I know I have already gone on about this, but it is really important.

LOOK AT THESE RESULTS FROM BOVINE CARTILAGE

When you see the results of Bovine Cartilage therapy, you can only be impressed. It was this report that gave me real hope that I could do something about my prostate cancer. The cancer the specialist said would kill me.

Listen to this and I quote from Doctor Prudden...

1. The disappearance of a very large rectal cancer with a demonstrated progressive normalisation obtained during treatment. Now take note of this my friend, it is important to you... this particular patient has been free of cancer now for **eighteen years** since the initial treatment!

2. The complete healing of a breast cancer ulcer of the **entire chest wall** after *failure of all standard therapy*. This patient was free of cancer for ten years until she died of an unrelated cause.

3. This case is particularly interesting to you. A presumptive cure of prostatic cancer, **metastatic to bones**, with complete normalisation of all blood values. That was one case that really inspired me. It brought home to me the critical fact that even if the cancer has leapt into my bones there was a definite hope of a cure.

4. The successful treatment of a widely metastatic cancer… got into the lungs and massively into the liver from its original source, the kidneys. The patient was a 76-year-old woman who lived for four years with normal lungs and gradually decreasing liver cancer. She died in a nursing home from an unrecognised rupture of an abscess.

   Now get this, my friend, at the autopsy **no trace of cancer was found in her body**. No trace of cancer remaining. Zilch.

These results are only three out of over a hundred similar stories. I spoke with the Australian manufacturer of Bovine Cartilage and he told me of many cases here in Australia where people with so-called incurable cancer had made remarkable recoveries.

Here's how you take Bovine Cartilage

Doctor Prudden found that giving patient nine grams of Bovine Tracheal Cartilage every day was the therapeutic dose. He gave it in three doses of three grams.

However, since then there has been a significant breakthrough. An Australian manufacturer has developed a technique to produce Bovine Cartilage in liquid form. This is pleasant tasting and seems to be just as effective as taking the powder form. It has the advantage that it is easier to take. And being liquid is more quickly absorbed into the bloodstream.

This is the Bovine I use myself. I am informed that Doctor Prudden has given his approval to the Australian breakthrough and is now using it himself with his patients instead of the powder.

But what about Shark Cartlilage?

Despite the fact over $7 million has been spent on research into the therapeutic effects of Bovine Cartilage it is not as well known as Shark Cartilage.

When you find you have cancer of whatever kind, you seem to become aware of different products to help. Shark Cartilage got a lot of publicity after a Cancer Convention in Canada. A paper was read on the good results with cancer of Shark Cartilage.

There are many people who will tell you that Shark Cartilage is superior to Bovine Cartilage in the treatment of cancer.

But let me give you all the facts so you can make an intelligent decision for yourself.

Again, I am quoting from Doctor Prudden's report...

There is a book by William Lane, Ph.D., called *Sharks Don't Get Cancer*, extolling the virtues of Shark Cartilage in cancer treatment. As a personal comment, I have never understood the title of this book. What has the fact that apparently sharks don't get cancer, as far as we know, got to do with Shark Cartilage helping cancer? It could be any part of the shark if you see a connection between the fact sharks don't get cancer and the shark itself.

This is not to say that Shark Cartilage doesn't help cancer. It is just my feelings about the title of the book.

Anyway, moving on. Doctor Lane makes a big case for Shark Cartilage to the disadvantage of other cartilages. But according to Doctor Prudden, this is because Doctor Lane assumes that only one factor is involved. Whereas, in fact, there are many factors involved. As Doctor Prudden puts it 'the positive cartilage effect is due not to one specific agent, but to the interaction of a complex array of molecular entities'.

However, whatever the virtues of taking Shark Cartilage let me tell you this... you have to take enormous amounts compared to Bovine Cartilage. And it's not the tastiest stuff in the world to take either!

The truth is that there has been nothing like the research on Shark Cartilage that there has been on Bovine Cartilage. Some long-term remissions with Bovine Cartilage have had a 19-year follow-up history and are considered presumptive cures.

Also, the quality of research of Bovine Cartilage is far superior to the research done on Shark Cartilage.

But forget all that, let's get down to cases.

It takes 9 grams of Bovine Cartilage a day to get a therapeutic result. With Shark Cartilage it takes from 70 to 100 grams! And that's a lot of powder to get into yourself, let me tell you!

Doctor David Williams, D.C., in one of his newsletters, comments that there are four significant disadvantages of Shark Cartilage that have little to do with the effectiveness or otherwise of it.

And Doctor Williams goes on to report that these disadvantages stop people from taking the full course of treatment. Or else, they take less than they should and it is therefore ineffective.

What are these four significant disadvantages?

It has a terribly fishy taste. The strong fishy smell. The high price. And finally, the difficulty of getting a consistent quality product. According to the newsletter, the quality of the Shark Cartilage can vary from manufacturer to manufacturer.

Let me illustrate this by telling you of a real case I know about. This person has what her medical advisors say is terminal cancer. It has gone from its original site to other places in her body.

She is taking Shark Cartilage but she has to take 100 grams a day. You have to see 100 grams to believe how much it is. This lovely lady persevered as long as she could but the smell, the taste and everything else proved too much.

She now has to take it as a suppository to get it into her.

So I much prefer to squirt some Bovine Cartilage into a glass of water. No nasty smell, no nasty taste and much much less expensive.

May I close this chapter by quoting from a book on Doctor Prudden's work by Alex Duarte O.D. Ph.D.:

What this in essence means is that we now have an effective and totally safe anti-cancer, anti-inflammatory, wound healing product that is simply non-toxic. Imagine a food that achieves far superior results compared to chemotherapy, radiation or surgery without mutilating or health-destroying side effects.

Hippocrates said it hundreds of years ago and it still holds true today: 'Let your medicine your food and your food your medicine'.

I will tell you where you can get Bovine Cartilage in Australia at the end of this book.

Isn't that exciting news?

Well, there are more exciting substances that your doctor doesn't know about. I will tell you more in the next chapter.

11 An incredible substance your doctor has never heard about! And it is a powerful anti-cancer agent!

In my work as a Naturopath I come across a lot of material not available to the public. I also subscribe to special newsletters and reports from other countries.

This is so I can keep up-to-the-minute with all the latest research and findings. I like to know what is going on out there!

Recently, I received a special report on new advances in healing and in this report were two important articles I would like to share with you.

They were both about a product you have probably never heard of... and neither will your doctor.

But both are critical in the battle against cancer of any form. That is important because whilst my book is mainly about prostate cancer there is a lot of information here that will benefit anyone with any other kind of cancer,

So let us go forward and have a look at this substance.

It is called 'Lactoferrin' and it does what may seem miraculous things in our bodies.

When you hear what lactoferrin does it is

An incredible substance... a powerful anti-cancer agent!

amazing that it is not a standard treatment for any sort of cancer. It does all the things we want a mighty anti-cancer treatment to do.

So what does it do?

Well, one of the things it does is to block cancer cell nourishment. It blocks off the supply of blood. This in turn causes the cancer to die. As I have mentioned, cancer cells need a lot of blood. So much so they set up their own network of blood vessels to make sure they get enough!

And lactoferrin stops this happening. Just like the troops cutting off the enemy's supply lines stopping food and ammunition getting through.

It also does something else quite remarkable. Lactoferrin activates DNA that launches immune responses. You will remember in Deepak Chopra's book how he said we had to get to the DNA to get it to bring cells back to normal. Well, lactoferrin is an agent in this department.

Lactoferrin creates natural antibodies to attack diseases that are trying to destroy us. This is like a general being able to call in extra troops to help him fight the battle. As a bonus, lactoferrin is also a potent anti-oxidant attacking and mopping up free-radicals.

The feeling with a lot of researchers is that we are on the brink of a bright future in medicine. They believe we are on the verge of a major medical breakthrough.

So much so that researchers are saying that because of the unique properties of lactoferrin, what the medical profession now think of as state-of-the-art treatment, such as radiation, antibiotics and chemotherapy, will one day seem as primitive and absurd as some of the earlier medical practices like blood-letting (where it was often said the patient died of the 'cure').

A lot more independent research is needed to see if lactoferrin can live up to its promise. If it does, then even fast spreading cancers may one day be as innocuous and manageable as a 24-hour bug! And wouldn't that be terrific.

WHAT THE HECK IS LACTOFERRIN ANYWAY?

Lactoferrin is an iron-binding protein that you get in your mother's milk. Yes, in what is called the 'colostrum'. This is your first armour against infection and disease. It is the first source of your immune system chemicals. It is the stuff your body uses to build its defence system.

And Nature in her wisdom puts this right where it is needed most... in a new-born baby's mouth, from Mum.

You will remember I have gone on about the immune system earlier in this book and the reason is it is so very important for our survival. Your immune system is constantly monitoring every cell in your body. It is making sure there is nothing there that shouldn't be there.

And if it discovers something there that shouldn't be there a healthy, strong immune system will launch a full-scale attack on the enemy within. It will send in the tanks, the rocket launchers, the flame-throwers — everything on hand to overwhelm the enemy. That is, if your immune system is healthy and strong.

Let us continue this discussion by changing tack.

HAVE YOU EVER WONDERED WHY A PREGNANT WOMAN'S BODY DOESN'T REJECT THE FOETUS?

I don't expect you have. But think about it!

A foetus in a woman's uterus is a foreign body. And your body throws out foreign bodies. It attacks them. This is the problem with organ replacement. The body rejects the transplant organ.

So why doesn't a woman's body reject the foetus?

The answer is because Nature automatically subdues the pregnant woman's immune system. And, of course, at this stage a pregnant woman shouldn't take lactoferrin because it would boost the immune system. And this would cause the woman to reject the foetus and a spontaneous abortion would happen.

But you know what happens as soon as the baby is born? That's right, the woman produces colostrum, and this restores her immune system. Now if that's not clever, I don't know what is!

But so clever is Nature the first milk the baby gets from Mum is pure colostrum. And this is packed with powerful immune chemicals to give the new-born baby the ability to resist attacks from predatory microbes and viruses.

This is a very cogent reason why mothers should breast feed their babies and resist the lures of advertising that tries to tell them formulas are just as good.

When I lived in Africa a major problem came up. African mothers have always breast fed their babies. Sometimes for as long as two years. Part of this was their belief that they couldn't get pregnant while breast feeding.

Anyway, thanks to clever promotions, a lot of African women were persuaded that the 'Western Way' of using formulas was better than the traditional way of breast feeding.

And thousands of little African infants died of starvation and disease. They no longer got the vital colostrum and to save money the African mothers diluted the formulas so they would last longer. Which shows that fashions are not necesssary healthy and can put survival at risk.

But back to lactoferrin and the immune system.

It is important to know that babies who do not get the colostrum, because the new Mum, for whatever reason decides to put the baby straight on to formula, tend to get sicker more often than babies breast fed by Mum.

But let's get on with lactoferrin. You have lactoferrin in most places where bugs love to go. The linings of your throat, your nose, tears and sweat. It is also found in some white cells called neurophils that surround and gorge on bacteria and viruses. But not enough.

People who are short of lactoferrin are always going down with illnesses. Illnesses you would expect them to fight off.

Lactoferrin has at least two specific immune-boosting functions.

It binds iron in your blood. This keeps it away from the cancer cells that love iron. They need iron to grow! And so do many bacteria, viruses and other nasties that get into our bodies. So by preventing them from getting the iron they need so urgently, they are destroyed.

But lactoferrin can release iron when necessary. And this makes lactoferrin a powerful anti-oxidant. You will remember that Free Radicals are generated by the billion all the time. They are responsible for our ageing and are also deemed to be responsible for diseases such as arthritis and cancer. So lactoferrin makes it hard for these Free Radicals, mopping them up like crazy.

But listen to this! Lactoferrin switches on the genes that launch your body's immune responses. It trips the switch. It presses the red button that causes the immune system to launch a massive response on the enemies within!

Research indicates that lactoferrin activates very specific strands of the DNA that turn on the genes that launch the immune response.

This is amazing!

And there is nothing else like it. Lactoferrin, as far as it is known, is a 'one off'. Incredible, isn't it?

You know, when I read information like this, I am amazed at the deep secrets locked in natural products. As Ruskin once remarked: 'The world does not lack wonders, it only lacks people who wonder'.

I liked the description of lactoferrin's action on cancer in the report I received from the Health Sciences Institute, Research Department: 'in effect, lactoferrin backs budding cancer cells into a corner... and sends out a signal to your white blood cells that says "It's over here! Come and get it!"'

At the end of this book I will let you know where you can buy lactoferrin.

Almost unbelievable news about lactoferrin and cancer!

Researchers in New York University and Harvard University have done extensive research on lactoferrin. And what they have discovered makes almost unbelievable reading!

First up, lactoferrin works much better than synthetic materials produced in some laboratory that bind free iron in the treatment for leukemia. This is breathtaking news for people with leukemia. I wonder how many have even heard of lactoferrin, never mind have the opportunity to try it out.

Lactoferrin appears to work against solid tumours.

But here is the most important action of all!

Lactoferrin appears to work against metastasis. This is the nasty way cancer cells migrate to other organs in the body. Lactoferrin works against this, the deadliest phase of cancer.

And this is the greatest fear of cancer sufferers. Will my prostate cancer get into my bones? Will my bowel cancer get into my liver?

And lactoferrin works to stop this happening!

Isn't that incredible news?

Just give a minute to read this case history...

One woman suffering from an aggressive lung cancer had been told her case was hopeless. She had lost weight dramatically and was down to a mere 85 pounds! Then she was lucky enough to come into the hands of one of the panel members at Health Sciences Institute and she was given lactoferrin.

At that time not only was the poor woman only 85 pounds she was nauseous, extremely weak and breathing with great difficulty.

Within weeks of beginning treatment, she began to regain her strength. She started to gain weight. Today, more than a year after she was told she was a hopeless case, she is still alive and going strong.

Her seemingly miraculous recovery is due largely to the healing power of lactoferrin.

You and I are mainly interested in lactoferrin as a help in curing prostate cancer but it has other startling properties.

It contains an anti-inflammatory molecule, which means it can help if you have arthritis.

It functions as an inhibitor of mammary cell growth. This means is would be great in the prevention or treatment of breast cancer.

It plays a role in ocular disturbances, which means that it may help with vision problems.

It is also showing potent anti-viral activity in reducing susceptibility to herpes infections.

All in all, an amazing substance. I hope you make this an important part of your weaponry against cancer or the risk of cancer.

It is recommended that people take lactoferrin daily whether they have a health threatening problem or not. Nothing but good can come from a powerful immune system in our polluted world!

Why haven't we heard about lactoferrin?

Simple! It can't be patented as it is a natural substance. This means there is no money in it for the big pharmaceutical companies. It really isn't worthwhile for them to spend the billions necessary to research the substance if they can't patent the results. There is no way for the company to get their money back. So one can hardly blame them for not spending a fortune researching lactoferrin.

However, it gets back to what I have said before. Your body can look after itself if you have a really powerful, hard-hitting, two-fisted immune system. Lactoferrin gives your body that power.

My thanks to the Health Sciences Institute for this information on lactoferrin.

I had to import Lactoferrin from America when I first found out about it. You couldn't get it in Australia...you can imagine how much that cost me. However, I would rather be the poorest man alive than the richest man in the cemetery.

The good news is you can now get it easily in Australia. All good health food shops and a lot of pharmacies now stock it under the brand name LactoMax. This is the one I use myself.

And that is what I do.

Can I share something with you?

Since I found out what at the time was incurable cancer, my life has changed. Well, what would you expect?

But it has changed for the better!

Because with all the vitamins and other supplements, my skin is clearer, I have more energy. I have that wonderful feeling of 'wellbeing'. This is almost a feeling of euphoria situated, in my case, around my solar plexus.

I truly appreciate every breath I take. And realising very personally that anger, jealousy and other negative emotions feed cancer, I am more relaxed and loving than I have ever been.

I recommend this to you most sincerely.

Let me explain something very important. I sincerely want this to get through to you, so forgive me for repeating myself.

Anxiety, hostility, anger are the most dangerous emotions in the world. It has been reported that these emotions cause stress that is an important component of at least 85% of all the illnesses we face in our society today.

And this includes cancer!

These emotions wear away your immune system. They damage delicate hormonal balance. Let me explain this a little further. These hormones include those from the adrenal gland, the pituitary gland, the thyroid gland and the thymus gland. And these glands are critical to your health.

If the flow of hormones from these glands become

unbalanced, you get sick! Very sick!

So keeping them in balance is vital to health. I told you how every thought creates a chemical and electrical response in your brain. The neurons in the brain create what are called 'neuro peptides'. And these are physical entities that can either uplift us or cast us down.

So keep your thoughts happy.

Always remember, my friend, you CAN beat cancer. It is not inevitable that an enlarged prostate will turn to cancer even though the orthodox opinion is an enlarged prostate is definitely 'pre-cancerous'. With the information in this book you can reduce the prostate back to normal and stop it becoming cancerous.

And if you don't have a prostate problem it would be wise to take notice of the advice in this book… the grim statistic is 60% of men will get a prostate problem. And it is my mission to reduce this figure as close to zero as I can.

In the next chapter let me introduce you to the wonderful,

12 How a little-known 200-year-old system of medicine can help you beat cancer!

almost magical world of Homeopathy and how it has helped me beat cancer.

When I studied Homeopathy over 15 years ago as part of my Naturopathic studies, I was amazed!

I found it hard to believe what I was reading. I remember writing in one of my answers to a test paper that 'I thought Homeopathy was 'magical'. To my amusement, my tutor wrote back and assured me that Homeopathy was not 'magical' and worked according to well researched science. Of course, I didn't think Homeopathy was magic. I knew it was a scientific, incredibly well-tested system of medicine. I meant the results seem almost magical — how well they worked.

But let me give you some brief examples of Homeopathy in action.

A lady came to see me with sore nipples from breast-feeding a lusty infant. I gave her the Homeopathic remedy, Arnica. She went out of the clinic and came back five minutes later.

'I can't believe this, but the pain has gone already. It went before I got back to my car which is just outside. Can Homeopathy work that quickly?'

Yes, it can. If you have the correct remedy for an acute condition.

Another case comes to mind. This delightful Brazilian lady had suffered with period pains that laid her up every month. She told me she felt as though her guts would drop out. She dreaded getting her monthly period because she went through agony every time.

So I gave her Sepia. And a month later I had this very excited lady on the phone: 'My period! She come and I don't even know it! Wonderful, wonderful. Now I say to my 'usband now, we 'ave the baby!'

Using Homeopathy, I have cured post-natal depression, eczema and a whole host of complaints. The only problem I have is that people usually come to me as a last resort. They have already been juiced up to blazes with drugs that didn't work and they come to me.

And I welcome them. Because quite often it is possible using Homeopathy and Clinical Nutrition to help them with their problem.

So what is Homeopathy?

The principles of Homeopathy were discovered by a Doctor Samuel Hahnemann in the late 1700s. He was a medical doctor and also a pharmacist. He wrote a lot of treatises on various pharmaceutical subjects.

He was quite disenchanted with orthodox medicine noting that more patients died from the attentions of the doctor than from the disease being attended to! As a Chemist he disapproved of the then new fad of using chemicals to attack disease. Whilst chemicals seemed to work more quickly than the traditional medical ways, the side effects were horrendous.

As I told you earlier, instead of using Sarsaparilla for treating the then epidemic proportions of syphilis, they used mercury. And he observed that what the experts called 'tertiary syphilis' was really advanced mercury poisoning.

In his experiments he discovered something startling.

He discovered that if you gave a susceptible healthy person a herb or a drug that caused him to become ill, that same substance would cure a sick person with the same symptoms.

Let me explain this a little further. It is not easy to grasp or to explain. But it is important to understand it.

Let us take a simple case. If I gave Aconitum to a person who was sensitive to Aconitum, he would get, among other things, a sore throat. By taking Aconitum, which taken as a herb is poisonous, the person would get a lot of symptoms, one of which could be a sore throat.

Now here is the mysterious part. The part doctors and others find especially difficult to grasp — if you give Aconitum to someone with a sore throat it will heal. And in many cases, heal very quickly.

The principle involved was called 'Similia Similibus Curanter' by Doctor Hahneman, which means 'like cures like'. Which again means that a Homeopathic medicine that will produce symptoms will cure diseases with similar symptoms.

The orthodox medical fraternity scoff at Homeopathy, mainly because they know nothing about it. The prejudice against Homeopathic principles is quite amazing. Just listen to this for a moment.

A French scientist found to his astonishment that water retained molecular powers even when there was no physical trace of any molecules. He did his experiments several times with the same results.

So he now got German scientists to do the same experiment and they got the same results. He also got some American scientists to test his theory and they too got the same results.

Excited, he sent a scientific paper on his findings to one of the most prestigious scientific journals, *Nature Magazine*.

And guess what? They refused to publish it. Why? Because they couldn't believe what they were reading even though the facts before them had been proven in different scientific experiments in different countries. This is censorship of science. And makes a mockery of the so-called 'scientific mind'.

Anyway, after a lot of protests, pressure and what have you, the editor finally agreed to publish the article. But even then, in his editiorial he said he didn't believe what had been published.

But Homeopathy has shown this to be true for 200 years.

You see, Homeopathy works at an energy level.

We Homeopaths believe that what is called 'disease' is not really disease at all. Well, come on folks, if it isn't disease, what the heck is it?

What we call disease is really our body's attempt to react to the agent causing us the problem. To give a simple example, I know it is difficult to understand, inflammation is not a disease. Inflammation is one of the body's reactions to a virus. Our bodies attempt to incinerate viruses, that is one reason we get a temperature and inflammation.

When the body recognises the protein of the virus, it secretes inflammatory agents like prostaglandins to generate inflammation. It is wise enough to realise that the best way to deal with a virus is to burn it up.

But often we mess it up by reducing the fever.

But getting back to Homeopathy...

Our bodies are activated by a chemical and electrical reaction. Drugs interfere with these reactions, causing side effects. Heroin, cocaine and even smoking interfere with these reactions in the brain. Death from an overdose of heroin is because the heroin interferes with the brain's ability to control breathing. The victim suffocates! Terrible, isn't it?

We are energy entities. Under the right conditions you would see people as flashing lights. Energy systems working at different capacities.

And Homeopathy is 'energy' medicine.

You may find what I am about to tell you unbelievable, but listen with an open mind. You remember I referred to Arnica earlier? Well, Arnica's full name is Arnica Montana. It is the Mountain Arnica, a member of the daisy family. Now get this, if you made a tea of the Arnica plant and drank it, do you know what would happen? You would be very ill and could die! Pretty violent stuff.

However, and this takes some believing. Arnica is wonderful for bruising, shock after an accident and all those symptoms one gets falling down mountains.

And Arnica in its natural state only grows above 1,500 feet. Herbalists believe it grows where its hidden powers are needed most. Fascinating stuff!

When Arnica is potentised according to Homeopathic principles, it is diluted beyond what is known as 'Avrogado's Law'. This says that beyond a certain point there is no longer any of the substance left in the liquid.

Now here is something to make you think.

All Homeopathic remedies go beyond the limits of Avrogado's Law!

This means that if you did an analysis of a Homeopathic medicine, nothing would show up!

And yet it still works! And works wonderfully well.

Isn't that amazing. You can see why I said I thought it was magic when I was first studying Homeopathy.

I have used Homeopathic medicines for post-natal depression, all sorts of skin problems, constipation, travel sickness, dogs with flea problems and cats with problems.

And if you would like to hear a really remarkable cure I effected, take a minute to read this.

One of our local veterinary surgeons phoned me with a critical problem. He had 17 greyhounds in his surgery and all had been injected accidentally with a lethal dose of an insecticide. I was surprised when the vet told me it was insecticide, but he assured me in normal doses this was all right.

And he went on to say: 'There is **no known antidote to it**!'

No known antidote and he wants to know if I can help. The reason he phoned me is because I had helped him Homeopathically in the past with small animal health problems with great success.

But there was no known antidote. The greyhounds were laying there very sick and would be dead before the day was out.

What could I do?

Well, this is what I did. I asked the vet to hurry down with some of the insecticide, whatever it was, that had poisoned the dogs. And this he did.

I then made up a Homeopathic medicine from the insecticide in a high potency. Remember, like cures like.

Later that day I got a most excited Vet on the phone telling me that 15 of the 17 dogs got on their feet after the first dose.

The end result was 15 dogs survived to race another day but the other two dogs were too far gone even for Homeopathy and they died.

May I say that the value of those dogs was over $70,000 and they were saved by a medicine costing only a few dollars.

Such is the 'magic' of Homeopathy when correctly prescribed.

CAN HOMEOPATHY HELP WITH CANCER?

There is one thing you should know. I may have already mentioned it. If I have, forgive me, but it bears repeating.

Naturopaths are forbidden in Australia to treat cancer patients!

This means that, officially, cancer patients only have medical treatments and when they fail, nothing! Because the medical profession has no more options to offer.

If they can't help you with drugs, surgery, chemo or

radiation, tough! You die!!

I heard that the reason was 'Naturopaths give "false hope"'. I explored this nonsense about false hope in an earlier chapter. The medicos believe that if a cancer patient goes to a Naturopath, the cancer could get out of control before they had a chance to do something to help.

And it is true that a lot of cancers, if detected early enough can be cured. But some can't!

So whilst I cannot treat cancer, there is nothing to stop me giving nutritional support. However, in most cases I see, it makes no difference.

Why? Because by the time they get to see me their doctors have given up on them. In other words, I get the hopeless cases!

I look after the despairing. I minister to those who have lost hope. I help the helpless.

But let me tell you, I have helped one man beat bowel cancer. He was to have surgery but by the time they came to do it the cancer had diminished to the degree no surgery was necessary.

I have two patients with what was deemed to be incurable cancer who are still going strong on Homeopathic medicines. They are plump, jolly and very happy. And look extrarordinary well!

I even have a canine patient. A much-loved old dog with cancer. He has outlived all expectations much to the delight of his loving owner.

I had one patient who phoned me from what was said to be her death bed. She only had weeks to live. Her voice was faint, I could hardly hear her. She told me she was too weak to get out of bed.

After listening to her I sent her some Homeopathic medicines. More in hope than expectation, I have to be honest to tell you.

Incredibly, after taking whole bottles of the medicine she phoned me again some weeks later. Her voice was much stronger and sounding a lot more lively.

I sent more Homeopathics down to her and she prospered. She was able to get out of bed and visit me. She put on weight and looked happy.

This was the person who only had weeks to live, bear in mind.

She lasted about two years before she died. She was able to travel and had a higher quality of life.

She stopped taking the Homeopathics and got into spiritual stuff. I am all for spiritual help, provided the patient does not abandon the more earthly remedies.

From my point of view, it was a great success. From deathbed to a much better life. From two or three weeks to two years. I honestly believe that had she kept on Homeopathics she could well have been here today.

So as you can see, Homeopathy can help cancer.

But it took me some time to remember this!

As I explained to you, when I discovered I had incurable prostate cancer, common-sense deserted me. In other words, I panicked!

And people who panic don't think clearly!

After I had got through the 'woe is me' stage I awoke up to the fact I had helped others with their cancer so it was time to help myself.

And I got down to cases and studied my own problem to find out how my knowledge of Homeopathy could help me. And now, to explain how it could help you.

Here's what I did to unleash the power of Homeopathy

By now you are familiar with my passionate belief in the power of our immune system. Given the materials it needs, I believe our immune system can deal with most problems that come up. Even with cancer!

So what did I have to do?

Well, I had to find out if Homeopathy could stimulate killer cell activity. Could Homeopathy do anything about my susceptibility to cancer?

You see, my Dad had bowel cancer and died of lung cancer. My grandmother died of cancer of the cervix. My brother had a large benign tumour removed from his armpit.

So I was definitely a candidate for cancer!

I am genetically susceptible according to the experts.

I explored the books to find the Homeopathic remedy that was specific for the prostate and had a record of helping prostate cancer.

And I am glad to tell you I was successful.

Now I am going to share that knowledge with you.

First, my susceptibility to cancer

Let me tell you something else that is hard to understand for a non-Homeopath. The higher the potencies, the stronger the medicine and the less of the original matter. So the meek inherit the earth. The weakest amount of the material produces the most dramatic results. That is ,when a high potency is called for.

So a 200 centesimal is stronger in action that a 30 (higher potencies are only prescribed where appropriate) even though there is much less of the original substance in the 200 strength.

But what is there, is a lot more healing energy!

So when I found the remedies that would help me I intended to use them in the higher potencies.

So the first remedy I looked for is called *carcinosinum*. This is what in Homeopathy they call a 'nosode'. It is actually made from diseased cancerous tissue. And you remember, like cures like, so someone with cancerous tissue is definitely susceptible to cancer.

So that was the remedy of first choice.

I believe this remedy builds up my resistance to cancer and overcomes my natural inherited susceptibility. This is the same remedy I give the old dog, with great success. I also always give it to cancer patients I am helping. The idea is to build up the natural resistant energies to cancer that we all have when healthy.

So this was my first remedy.

My next one is T4. I can make up a remedy called T4 and what this does is activate the T4 'killer' cells in my body. This boosts my defence system enormously. The more active the T4 cells the better chance I had of beating the cancer that was threatening my life.

So this was my second remedy.

Behind your breast bone you have a gland called the Thymus Gland. It was once thought that this gland withered away as we grew older. This was because when autopsies were done, the gland was small and withered looking.

But now it has been discovered that the cart was being put before the horse. It was because the Thymus was withered and small that the person got sick and died. A healthy person has a full-sized Thymus. But all the observations had been made on sick people.

So the conclusion that as we grow older our Thymus shrivels up is not true. The other deduction, also incorrect, was that as the Thymus shrivelled up as we grow older, we don't need it!

But, of course, it doesn't shrivel as we age in healthy people, and we do need it.

Let me give you an important little tip.

As an example let me say this, I am extremely allergic to tobacco smoke. It gives me a headache and makes my eyes water and I feel nauseous. Much like you felt when you puffed on your first fag!

But if I tap my chest vigorously the feeling goes away. This is because by tapping my chest I activate my Thymus gland. This in turn boosts my immune system and bingo! I feel better.

I have verified this myself and watched other practitioners verify it too. It is easily done. In something called 'Kinesiology' you test muscle strength. The subject extends his or her arm and the practitioner gently presses it downwards.

He notes how much resistance he gets. Then he asks the subject to hold a substance to which he or she is allergic. And do you know what happens?

The subjects go weak.

Now you can do this with, in my case, tobacco. Test my arm and it is strong. Give me a cigarette to hold and my arm goes weak. Take away the cigarette and my arm still tests weak.

But here is something very interesting. If I tap my chest two or three times and then test my arm again, guess what? Yes, it tests strong.

Kinesiology is very accurate. I use it a lot to test people for allergies. And it also reveals quite clearly that if you activate the Thymus the body gets strong.

This will work for you too. Try it on someone.

Here's a simple experiment for you. Get a friend or your partner to hold out one arm. You face your partner and place one hand on your partner's shoulder, over the deltoid muscle.

Now with your other hand gently try to depress the extended arm.

Explain to your partner that this is not a trial of strength. That is why you will find the experiment works better if you use a female partner. Too many blokes think it is something like arm wrestling!

You should find the arm quite steady.

Now ask your partner her name. Her real name. She will tell you her name and her arm will still test strong.

Now here is something quite mysterious. Ask you partner to give you a false name. And her arm will immediately go weak.

Your body knows when you are lying.

Isn't that amazing?

And I have used this method to detect the fact that the Thymus is working.

Which leads me to my third remedy. Yes, you've guessed it. Thymus. I make up Homeopathic Thymus to stimulate my Thymus Gland to release lots of aggressor cells to leap to my defence!

As I keep saying, it is a marvellous and mysterious world in which we live. That is why it does not do to believe we have all the answers on anything.

Humanity reminds of a little boy who wandered into a vast library. A library as big as the universe itself. Rows and rows of books, billions and billions of them. The little boy pulls down one volume, reads the introduction and believes he knows the contents of the cosmic library!

That is about the state of our much vaunted knowledge. There is so much we don't know. It doesn't do to be arrogant when it comes to knowledge of what goes on in the universe. And I am not talking about astronomy alone!

There are Cosmic Laws we don't know about. But every day we pay the price for our ignorance. It is a bit like breaking the speed limit because you didn't see the sign. You didn't realise you were doing anything wrong.

Tell that to the cop when he pulls you over!

You will still get a ticket.

And I believe it is the same with the Cosmic Mind. There are laws we don't know about but we still pay a price for our ignorance. Unhappiness, disease, misfortune, lost hopes, poverty... the list is almost endless.

So it doesn't do for doctors to knock Homeopathy simply from ignorance. They say there is no bad Homeopathy, only some bad Homeopaths who do not prescribe the right medicine in the right potency.

Now I have my Carcinosinum to balance my susceptibility to cancer. I have my T4 to activate my attacker cells and my Thymus to stimulate my Thymus to release more attacker cells.

So now I decided to do something about the prostate itself.

And the remedy of choice here is Sabal Serrulata. You have met Sabal before under another name, Saw Palmetto. But I intended to take Saw Palmetto as a herb and as a Homeopathic medicine too.

And so there it is. That is what I take. And let me tell you, one reason so much misinformation is given about Homeopathy is because it is very inexpensive. It cannot be patented. High prices cannot be charged like they are for drugs.

Homeopathic medicines have been on trial for 200 years, unlike modern drugs. They have been tested on human beings, not animals. No rabbits, dogs, white rats have suffered. No chimpanzees, only humans have proved these remedies.

So they are well tested. Perfectly safe. You can take them with the greatest confidence.

There are prohibited substances that specialists claim can help cancer. One is Laetrile. This is from apricot kernels. At one time you could buy this quite freely in Australia.

That is until they discovered it had a percentage of cyanide in it!

Shock, horror. Let's save the public from themselves. I am always suspicious when someone is doing something for my good, without asking my permission, so it was banned!

You can get Laetrile treatment in clinics in Mexico but not anywhere else that I am aware of. But you can get it Homeopathically.

There are nosodes for specific cancers, by the way. I have them for breast cancer, colon cancer and even lung cancer. I have never used them in my practice so I can't really tell you how effective they are.

But I can tell you that when properly prescribed Homeopathy seems to work just like 'magic'… no matter what my tutor says!

In the next chapter I will give you a rundown on various remedies that are seen as useful in treating cancer.

13 Healers unknown to your doctor

When I researched prostate cancer in depth to help myself I was quite astonished at the number of alternative options open to any cancer sufferer. And to those who are determined not to get it!

Unfortunately, the great majority of people with cancer go to their graves unaware that there are so many options they could have taken advantage of to improve their lot.

And equally distressing to me is the number of people who get cancer who needn't have got it. Just by following the guidelines in this book I believe it is possible to go through life without suffering the misery of cancer.

The key is knowledge. By reading books like this one, you have your eyes opened. You suddenly realise there are heaps you can do easily to prevent yourself going through all that suffering.

I tell you what, I wish I had known what I know now when my dear Dad had lung cancer. He received no treatment other than morphine to kill the pain. In the end, even morphine didn't work and he died in agony. Had I known then what I know now, I am sure things would have been different.

That is another reason for writing this book. I passionately want anyone with any kind of cancer to realise that their doctor does not know everything. There are a lot of things that can be done in conjunction with standard cancer treatment.

Look at vitamins. Vitamin C in particular. For anyone on radiation or chemotherapy, Vitamin C is a godsend. Taking up to 20 grams a day can prevent the hair falling out and reduce the nausea associated with these treatments.

What is interesting about taking such a large amount of Vitamin C is that normally that amount would give you diarrhoea but in this case it doesn't. Why? Because your body is using every single atom of it..

Vitamin B1 helps to prevent cancer by detoxifying various carcinogenic chemicals. Vitamin B3 has a major role in the prevention and treatment of cancer. B6 retards the growth of certain cancers.

Vitamin A and its precursor Beta-Carotene are essential in any treatment or prevention of cancer.

Vitamin A helps to prevent prostate cancer by strengthening the mucous membranes inside the prostate gland.

Beta-Carotene reduces the risk of prostate cancer. A good reason to eat lots of carrots, pumpkins and all red and yellow fruits and vegetables.

We hear a lot these days about the so-called toxicity of Vitamin A. Can I take a moment to put this in perspective. In Australia the maximum tablet amount is 5,000 i.u. And a warning notice is on every container telling people that overdosing on Vitamin A can cause birth defects.

This is because one person took more than the stated amount, which in those days was 10,000 i.u. (and had been at that level for zonks!) and sadly she had a malformed birth.

However, as a lady doctor pointed out, by far more birth

defects are caused by lack of Vitamin A than were ever caused by it. Cleft palate in some cases has been linked to a Vitamin A deficiency in the mother.

Your liver can store 500,000 i.u. of Vitamin A. There have been countless people on mega doses of Vitamin A — 150,000 a day, under medical supervision, without ill effects.

So where cancer is concerned, my belief is to get into the Vitamin A in loads. I take 50 or more mgs of Vitamin A every day. That is about 80,000 i.u. I see this as a vital part of my cancer treatment.

Just look at this list of cancer sufferers who usually have low levels of Vitamin A. Bladder Cancer, Breast Cancer, Cervical Cancer, Lung Cancer, Pharyngeal Cancer, Prostate Cancer, Skin Cancer, Stomach Cancer and Cancer of the Testicles (a fast-growing cancer today).

An impressive list, isn't it?

It is interesting to note that most cancer victims are low in Vitamin A. It would seem sensible to take Vitamin A as a cancer preventative. It is also a necessary part of an effective immune system.

So get into the Vitamin A and Beta-Carotene!

Vitamin D, which often comes with Vitamin A, has a valuable contribution to make to reversing enlargement of the prostate and also cancer.

It is important to take only the prescribed amount of Vitamin D because excessive Vitamin D can cause an irrreversible build up of calcium in the body. It is fine as long as you stick to the recommended dosage.

HERBS THAT HELP CANCER

In addition to the other herbs I have already told you about, there are a couple more that have a record of helping cancer.

The first is Pau d'Arco.

Pau d'Arco is a remarkable herb from South America. Doctors there have been reporting dramatic cases of tumours shrinking, pain easing and hopeless cancer conditions going into complete remission.

And how many folks do you think have even heard of Pau d'Arco? Not many, I can tell you.

It was discovered in 1966 by an Argentinian Botanist, Doctor Theodore Mayer. So it is a recent addition to the Herbal Defence System.

Pau d'Arco successfuly treated lesions in breast cancer and despite the opinion of the American Cancer Institute, research has shown that Pau d'Arco is essentially non-toxic at moderate levels.

From our point of view (yours and mine), the South American doctors' reports which revealed that by using Pau d'Arco they have seen tumours shrinking, pain disappearing and patients declared 'terminal' going into complete remission, is wonderful news.

It just goes to show how little is really known about treating cancer. I would like to see a lot more of the cancer research dollar going into proving the efficacy of the herbs, vitamins and other supplements I am discussing here with you,

It would be refreshing to see more publicity given to telling people how they can take simple steps to prevent degenerative diseases like cancer. This book is my contribution to getting the message out there, a simple message: 'You can prevent yourself from getting cancer'.

THE HUMBLE BUMBLE BEE HAS A PART TO PLAY TOO!

It is my belief that everything in this Universe has its place. Everything serves some purpose. It may be that we do not know what that purpose is, but that doesn't mean it doesn't have a purpose. It only means we don't know what it is!

And it is a source of wonder how many, very ordinary, everyday sources of helpful medicines there are to help suffering humanity.

Take Bee Pollen, as an example.

Scientific research has shown that Bee Pollen increases the number of cancer retarding red corpuscles erythrocytes by as much as 25 to 30%. And this helps our body to resist cancer.

I am a great believer in preventing cancer. Had I known a few years ago what I know now, I would never have got prostate cancer at all. And that would have saved me a lot of terrible anguish.

I sincerely hope by writing this book I will spare other men the misery I went through.

Amino acids: building blocks to health!

Your body is built from amino acids. They are the basic building blocks of your body.

But while we need aminos to build muscle, tissue and other visible signs of a body that is growing, there are amino acids that have specialised functions.

And that is what I want you to find out right now.

Methionine is an amino acid commonly used in fat metabolising formulae. It is excellent for the liver. I have prescribed Methionine often for people with Hepatitis. People with poor liver function.

I have had great results with it for lowering cholesterol levels. This is because around 80% of your cholesterol is made in your liver. Improve liver function and it stops over-producing cholesterol.

But Methionine has some other, not so well-known qualities.

One is that it slows down male pattern baldness. A cream made from Methionine and Cysteine helped restore hair in 75% of the people treated. Methionine and Cysteine taken together help hair growth.

I give you this information as a bonus!

Methionine can a also reduce the craving for alcohol, which could be good news for some. Especially if they have prostate cancer. Alcohol goes straight to the prostate.

People with prostate enlargement or cancer should avoid alcohol. You will find increasd difficulty in urinating after drinking... at a time when you have more than usual amounts to release.

Heavy metals in the body have been associated with cancer. And Methionine binds to these metals and takes them out of the body.

Here is something important. Methionine in large amounts is toxic. Also, in large amounts, it takes calcium out of the body contributing to osteoporosis.

So do not go beyond the recommended dose, at which level it is perfectly safe to take.

Ornithine, Glycine and Cysteine all help to elevate the immune system. Anything that boosts the immune system is good news for cancer sufferers. As it is good news for people with a lot of other diseases. And for people who don't want any problems.

HAVE YOU EVER HEARD OF CO ENZYME Q 10?'

Even though a lot of people may never have heard of Co Enzyme Q 10, it is essential for health. In fact, if you had no Co Enzme Q 10 in your body you would be in BIG trouble.

It is necessary for the production of energy. It is essential for a healthy heart.

Have you noticed something? People with high energy levels are usually very healthy. Now which came first? Was it because they have high energy levels that they are healthy or is it because they are healthy that they have high energy levels?

The answer is... who cares?

High energy is essential for good health. High energy goes with wellness. High energy goes with low stress. When you have lots of energy you can cope with catastrophes that floor the people with low energy.

What is the picture you have of someone who is sick?

Someone with a downcast expression, a look of pain and very low energy! We see people with high energy levels as healthy.

'I wish I had your energy' is a common cry.

Well, Co Enzyme Q 10 gives that priceless energy.

I have seen people do a test on an ergomatic machine before and after taking Co Enzyme Q 10. And the difference was amazing.

After taking Co Enzyme Q 10, even people over 60 turned in much better figures. They were able to perform for much longer. It was noticeable to them as well as the measuring device.

So boosting the ability of cells to put out energy can only help.

I take Co Enzyme Q 10, and as a comment, people often ask me where do I get my energy from!

Hey! Take care. The water you drink may be killing you!

You know, when you look at a glass of water out of your tap it looks great. It sits there sparkling in the sunlight. Mmmm... let's get some!

But the first thing, perhaps the only thing you notice, is the smell of chlorine.

People often tell me they don't need a water purifier because they boil their water. In the suburbs? They boil the water! Why do they do that?

I explain to them that boiling the water is a waste of time. There are no bugs in the water. No bug can live in all that chlorine. That's why they put the chlorine in it. To kill the bugs.

You see, chlorine is a bleach. It is a poison.

And chlorine depresses your immune system.

And it is a strong immune system that will work to prevent you getting cancer or other health problems you do not want.

And your drinking water is full of it.

Let's be honest here. To be healthy, and that is surely everyone's goal, we have to be very careful what we take into our body.

There is an old saying that goes something like this: 'If you want to know the result of all your yesterdays, look in the mirror!' We are the result of what we think, what we eat and what we drink.

We create our own future.

And I dearly want your future to be free of disease. I want your future to be one of glowing good health for all your days.

Getting back to the water in your tap. It also can have mercury and lead. These are both poisonous and there is no 'safe' level.

If that isn't bad enough you can have pesticides, herbicides, fertilizers and other farm chemicals in your water. That is because in today's agri-business, chemicals play a large part. And they run off into the water supply. But you can't see or detect them!

So filtering water, before drinking it, makes sense. In our home we only ever use filtered water for any use where the water comes into our mouths.

We use it for making tea and coffee. We use it for making soup. We use it for steaming our vegetables. We only drink filtered water.

And I urge you to do the same.

Oh, here is a totally irrelevant piece of information. It is relevant to staying healthy and not getting prostate problems. Men who have a vasectomy are much more likely to get prostate problems than men who have not had one. Men who have their vasectomy when less than 35 years old are particularly at risk.

I thought I would just throw that in.

WHAT HELPS TO CURE CANCER HELPS TO PREVENT IT!

It is important to stress that the herbs, the amino acids, the vitamins, the supplements that help relieve cancer are vital if you want to be sure you never get it.

When you think that cancer is one of the fastest growing forms of killer diseases in our society it makes sense to take steps to protect yourself.

When I first thought about writing this book, I had two objectives. One was to help anyone with prostate or other form of cancer. But even more so, I desperately want to make sure that as many people as I can reach with this book learn how to PREVENT it.

I write in the first two chapters about the horrors of finding out I had cancer. This was done not to wear my agony on my sleeve. It is intended to let you know what you too can go through if you don't take steps NOW to be sure you don't become a victim.

When you realise that something like 80% of all men will get a prostate problem you realise the wisdom of making sure you are not one of them.

But getting back to little-known anti-cancer prevention substances. In Australia few people have heard of Melatonin. Anyway, even if they have heard of it, they can't buy it. It is not to be seen anywhere.

This contrasts with America where every vitamin store has a large display of Melatonin by the entrance. You can't miss it!

Now most people take Melatonin because it is seen as great for insomnia. Can't get off to sleep? Take Melatonin and you will!

But what is not generally recognised is Melatonin has other great properties. It promotes the release of chemicals that work synergistically to prevent cancer.

If, like me, you are genetically prone to cancer you will be interested to learn that Melatonin prevents genetically-related cancers.

So it makes Melatonin an important part of any regime to prevent cancer of any sort, including prostate.

How bitter melons prevent cancer!

I have heard of bitter lemons, but I had never heard of bitter melons. That is, until I went to America with my friend, Frank Caruso.

We went into a vitamin shop and it was stacked from floor to ceiling with containers of bitter melon tablets. We couldn't believe it!

It turned out that he was a wholesaler who also sold his one product to the public. And that product was bitter melon.

He assured us that bitter melon was set to sweep across America. I don't know if it ever did. It certainly has not yet made it here in Australia.

But bitter melon is very helpful in preventing cancer. This is because unripened bitter melon increases the number of helper T cells.

And you will remember that it is T cells that demolish cancer cells. So having plenty of them around is insurance against cancer as they can launch an attack before the cancer gets a hold.

So I expect that people in America take heaps of these tablets to make sure they don't get cancer!

THE PUZZLE OF WHY A CHINESE PROVINCE HAD SO MUCH CANCER

Authorities in China were worried.

In one of their provinces the rate of cancer of the throat was far higher than the national average. It seemed that people were doomed to get this malady and to perish.

So a team of researchers was sent in to see if they could discover what was causing this terrible problem.

Well, it wasn't radiation. There were no nuclear plants within hundreds of miles. And there hadn't been an accident or release of radioactive materials. So that was out.

It didn't run in families. Whole villages randomly had people suffering and dying from this cancer.

So what could it be?

Eventually they narrowed the search down and found it was the soil. The soil in this province lacked Selenium. And without Selenium cancer was able to get hold of its victims.

Once the authorities supplemented the soil with Selenium, the cancers dropped back to the national average!

Now this raises an interesting point.

Most of the soils in the Western world are deficient. Because of years of mono-farming, drenching the soil with fertilizers, herbicides and pesticides, most soils are deficient. In fact, in many cases, without the chemicals applied by the tonne, nothing would grow.

In Australia people selling vitamins, for example, are prohibited from telling people that because of depleted soil they would be well advised to take a multi-vitamin/mineral tablet every day. I guess this would upset the agricultural lobby and the chemical industry.

But the Chinese experience demonstrates how by being short of just one vital element there can be disastrous consequences!

Selenium protects the body by stimulating the anti-carcinogenic actions of phagocytes. The cells in your immune system that play a vital part in your body's defence system.

Selenium in large amounts is toxic. But it would have to be very large amounts. Taken as indicated on the container it is fine and can only be helpful,

In Australia you cannot buy Selenium in tablet form. You could, years ago. But not today. Some person took a whole heap ignoring the instructions and got sick, as you would expect. So the authorities banned it.

Good job they don't do this with motor cars. Some idiot drives a car into a pole so they ban that make of car. Could you imagine it? Well, that's exactly what they do if some fool overdoses on a supplement such as Selenium.

Happily, you can now get Selenium as a food. You get it in powder form along with vitamins A, C and E. So you not only have a great cancer preventative, you also have a great anti-oxidant booster too!

THIS IS A GREAT ANTI-CANCER FORMULA

A very popular formula is called Essiac. This is the name of the inventor of this formula, whose name is Caisse. And

Selenium is now available over the counter in Australia

Essiac is Caisse spelled backwards.

The major herb in this formula is Sheep Sorrel. In most Herbals you will find that Sheep Sorrel is given as a great skin remedy. Very helpful for someone with Psoriasis, for example.

But Sheep Sorrel is also a great defence against cancer. In the case of the Essiac formula, Sheep Sorrel is the major ingredient, as I said. It is only part of the total formula.

However, in my cancer prevention research, Sheep Sorrel is seen as a very useful herb to combat cancer and to prevent it.

So I recommend it to you.

South America to the rescue!

Have you ever heard of a herb called Pau d'Arco? You can find this in some vitamin stores sitting there on the shelf. But I'd like to bet that very few of the people shopping there are aware of this herb's power.

Now, I've got something important to tell you... this herb has a reputation among a lot of doctors in South America that will amaze you. Doctors there are reporting dramatic cases of tumours shrinking, pain disappearing... and get this, hopeless cases of cancer going into complete remission. I am not just talking about prostate cancer here. But all kinds of cancer.

When we think of herbs, we usually think of some bonnetted lady peering out of her thatched cottage lovingly looking at her herb garden. We usually have a picture reminiscent of lavender and lace... mental pictures of another century.

So it may come as a bit of a surprise to discover that the potent powers of Pau d'Arco were only discovered in the late 1960s. Your great grandmother certainly did not have Pau d'Arco in her armoury of herbs!

To be honest, Pau d'Arco is not really a herb at all. It comes from the inner bark of a tree that rejoices in the odd name of the Tabeluia tree.

Believe it or not, but Pau d'Arco was tested 20 odd years ago by the National Cancer Institute in America and found to be successful in helping breast cancer... But they did nothing with the information. Why not? Because they thought it might be toxic as some people became nauseous... they ought to look at people who are on chemotherapy, for goodness sake!

Later research has proven that Pau d'Arco is non-toxic at moderate dose levels.

Now South American doctors are reporting exciting results with Pau d'Arco... They claim it has been the main cause of almost unbelievable cases of tumours shrinking,. pain disappearing and patients once diagnosed as terminal going into remission.

Of course, there is only one way to find out and that is to try it for yourself. You can get Pau d'Arco in almost any Health Food shop that stocks supplements.

Follow the manufacturer's instructions on the pack.

Some call this 'The Mediterranean Miracle Herb'

It's a funny thing with we humans. We are surrounded by miracles large and small but we seldom notice them. We need fire and smoke, crashing of thunder, visions and other stage effects to believe anything is really some kind of miracle.

But the herbs and supplements I have told you about are all miracles in their own way.

The other thing about is that we see things without seeing them, if you know what I mean. For years we have seen how Mediterranean people thrive on Olive Oil as a main ingredient in their diets. But apart from recommending Olive Oil on our salads we have not drawn any other conclusions.

That is... until now.

Super bugs are here... the modern plague!

You have read in your newspapers frightening articles on the arrival of the 'super bugs'. These are microbes that are no longer affected by our most powerful antibiotics. Microbiologists are warning of a return to the dark days when, if you got pneumonia, you either lived or died. The doctors had no medicine, no drugs, to help you.

And they say these days will soon be upon us again.

They say the cause is that doctors have been far too free in handing out antibiotics for the most trivial of complaints. The germs reproduce at such an incredible rate they are able to breed a new species of bug... a bug that laughs at our antibiotics. What is worse, the number of these bacteria is growing by the day.

So what will happen when doctors are powerless to help with their once powerful drugs?

The medical opinion is 'Tough'... we will be back in the dark ages.

The herbal view is that we will, at last, realise the power lying there in herbs. Remember, all doctors were herbalists at one time... chemical drugs are the new kids on the block!

THE HUMBLE OLIVE LEAF COULD BE JUST WHAT WE ARE LOOKING FOR!

Olive leaves contain something called 'Calcium Elenolate'... and this is big medicine according to the reports I have examined. As you have gathered, I am a great believer in building up the health of the 'host' where cancer is concerned. And this really applies to any disease state someone may find themselves in.

Boosting the immune system, getting the patient into as good a physical shape as we can, is good medicine.

You remember how the Naturopath Hulda Clark in her best-selling books on Cancer and health promotes the view that parasites are often a hidden and unsuspected cause of ill health and cancer? She tells us how important it is to rid ourselves of parasites that grow in our bodies.

And Olive Leaf extract is deadly to parasites...

Glycoproteins are very important here but so is the humble Olive Leaf.

What is incredible is Olive Leaf extract has been known for over 100 years for its remarkable medicinal qualities.

Have you noticed Olive Leaf Extract anywhere on your travels?

No, and neither have I... until quite recently.

Olive Leaf extract was used for treating Malaria successfully and with no side effects. It was said to be more effective than quinine... but no longer used... strange, isn't it?

It is quite shocking that we have had this marvellous substance available for all that time but nothing has been done about it.

But things are changing.

Olive Leaf extract and other natural substances are seen to be our saviours in a world where superbugs become the 'untouchables'.

Just listen to this list of specific things Olive Leaf extract will address...

It stops viruses from growing by interfering with certain amino acid production that are vital for viruses and even bacteria to grow. It does something else too... it stops viruses from doing their number on us. It inactivates the little horrors.

Here is something really dramatic... Olive Extract (the Calcium Elenolate factor) can actually get into our cells and shut down the viruses' ability to reproduce. This is startling information. Just think about the importance of this.

Olive Leaf extract,. according to the papers I have studied, directly stimulates the immune cells that devour viruses and bacteria. Stimulated by Calcium Elenolate, the phagocytes (as they are called) have a field day chewing up all the bacteria and viruses in sight.

This is a real-life **natural** antibiotic.

And what is great about it is that because it is natural and not made in some chemical factory, each leaf is slightly different and the bugs cannot adapt to it.

Also, as it is a natural substance, Olive Leaf extract has a much wider range of actions than man-made antibiotics.

Olive Leaf extract has a built-in-bonus. It is excellent for supporting circulation, normalising blood pressure, prevents hardening of the arteries and even normalises blood sugar levels.

Definitely something to look into... and available right now either in your local Health Food store or from your Health Professional.

It is a substance I would recommend for not only boosting the immune system but also for acting as a mighty second string to it.

This is not just for someone with a prostate problem of any kind but for everybody interested in health. Certainly it fits in with my philosophy of building the host, the patient himself or herself, to enable them to resist and cure disease.

YOUR BOWEL IS IMPORTANT TOO

Constipation is bad for the prostate.

Straining to pass stool brings unwelcome pressure on your prostate. So it is sensible to be sure you can pass the waste matter easily and without strain.

There is a lot of emphasis these days on getting enough fibre into our diets. A lot of people rush out and grab a bag of Wheat Bran to put on their cornflakes.

But Wheat Bran is not for everyone. For a lot of people it is too rough. And quite a lot of people are allergic to wheat.

Better to use Rice Bran, Oat Bran, Pysillium Husks or Slippery Elm Bark because these are gentle fibres that will keep things moving without strain.

14

Here's how to avoid the devastating effects of prostate surgery... The secrets to not getting a prostate problem... ever!

I wrote this book for three separate people.

And I know you are one of those three!

Who are they? Well, the first is someone who does not have a prostate problem right now. And sensibly, doesn't want one either! This person wants to know as much as possible about the prostate so he can make sure he never has a problem.

If this is you, you are exceptionally wise.

The second person is the man who knows he has a problem. He knows he is suffering from Hypertrophied Prostate. The options he has been given are not cheery. Drugs and quite often, surgery.

You have been told that they can 'ream' out your prostate gland to made it smaller and take the pressure off your bladder. It may have been suggested that you take drugs to reduce the size of the prostate. You may have been encouraged to take antibiotics 'in case there is infection in the bladder'.

All in all, you are not very happy with the options. The prospects of surgery fill you with foreboding. You've heard a lot of bad reports. Incontinence, unlucky patients having to wear special waterproof underwear and other humiliating effects. You do not want to be part of this.

So you are sensibly looking for other ways to bring down the size of your prostate. And in this book you will have found them. In this chapter I am simply going to summarise them for you in a handy form.

And finally, you have prostate cancer. I trust you have found hope from my experience. You now realise there are lots of options open to you. You can take steps to save your life.

Do not accept the death-sentence kind of options handed down. Read this book several times, make notes, and then DO IT. Do as I have suggested and you WILL WIN. I have no doubt about it.

So you don't have a prostate problem... And don't want one!

So let me first sum everything up for you if you are the reader who has read a bit about prostate problems and doesn't want anything to do with the problem.

First up, get rid of false modesty. Go and see your doctor.

Let me re-emphasise something very important.

False modesty can KILL you.

Early discovery of a problem makes certain it will never get to something really serious.

Go every year to your doctor and have a digital examination of your prostate gland. You will find all your fears of embarrassment were groundless. Your doctor does these examinations every day. They are routine. Please, do yourself a favour. Go every year and have a digital examination.

It takes only five minutes and they could be the most important five minutes of your life. Breast cancer in women is coming down and it is directly due to the publicity given to breast examination.

More women than ever before are having regular breast examinations. And as a result, the number of breast cancer cases and deaths is dropping.

So go. Phone and make an appointment RIGHT NOW. Don't put it off. DO IT!

GET A PSA TEST DONE WHILE YOU ARE THERE

A digital will not always reveal you have prostate cancer. My examination showed only a slight enlargement, even though 60% of my prostate gland was cancerous.

So get a PSA. You will remember that PSA stands for Prostate Specific Antigen and reveals if you have cancer of the prostate.

The test involves the doctor taking a sample of your blood and sending it to a pathology laboratory for testing. The results come back in a couple of days.

Do this every year. In the case of cancer, prevention is infinitely preferable to attempts at cure!

BE ALERT FOR SIGNS OF A PROSTATE PROBLEM

Continuing.

Be alert to signals that a problem is developing. Ignore these signals at your peril! They are flashing red danger signals. Listen to your body.

If you notice that you are getting up more often during the night to go to the toilet. If you are getting up two and three times a night where before you slept right through... Watch out!

An early warning sign is this business of having to get up. The reason is your prostate is enlarging and blocking off the exit from your bladder.

When you go to the toilet you are not emptying your bladder completely.

Another sign is the flow. If you notice that the flow of urine is not what it was... look out! When you were younger you can pee over a wall, easy! If your flow now is diminished... If you find it is taking you longer to empty your bladder... If you are first in the urinal and last to leave... watch it! This is another clear sign something is wrong.

If you have any pain passing water, see your doctor immediately. If you have burning anywhere along the tract — before, during or after urinating — get to the doctor.

Famous last words are 'it will go away'. It doesn't!

Another unwelcome sign of a prostate problem affects our sex life. We never like to admit we have sexual problems. But that doesn't make them go away.

If you find that these days you cannot maintain an erection... then go and see your doctor. This is another prostate problem sign.

A not so obvious sign is when you have had a few drinks you find it difficult to empty your bladder. You are bursting but can only pass urine by the drop when you want to pass it by the bucketful!

This is another warning signal. You are in danger. It is another flashing red light. Go and get an examination!

Terrific. Everything is just fine!

Congratulations. I am delighted everything is fine. But follow the steps I have outlined above.

Here are the other things you need to do to make sure you never have the misery and suffering of a prostate that has gone haywire.

Take zinc every night before you go to bed.

This is critical. It is very important. Your prostate needs zinc to keep healthy. There is no doubt about this.

Secondly, take Saw Palmetto. This herb is just about the best there is for a healthy prostate. This and zinc are cheap insurance, believe me.

To be healthy you must have a gung ho immune system. Your immune system must always be in a state of red alert. Able to take on anything stupid enough to face it.

So take Grape Seed, Vitamins A, C and E. These will boost your immune system and keep it toned up.

As good health is critical, do your best to eat a healthy diet.

If you don't think diet is all that important consider these facts. These statistics refer to colon cancer, but could just as easily refer to almost any kind of cancer, including prostate.

'A study of 1,225 patients with colon cancer and 728 with rectal cancer found something of importance to you and me. It was noted that there were significant trends of increasing risk of colecteral cancer with an increased consumption of bread and cereal dishes, potatoes, cakes and desserts. And also refined sugar. Intakes of fish, raw and cooked vegetables, fruits other than citrus showed a reduced risk of cancer.'

These figures could apply to most cancers. High fat diets are often implicated in prostate cancer. As is high alcohol consumption.

Eating a low fat, high fibre diet makes a lot of sense if you want to avoid disease. And I am not just talking about cancer.

There are a lot of diseases directly attributed to poor diet.

Arthritis, circulation and arterial problems. Heart attacks. Strokes. Diverticulitis... loads of them!

So eat a healthy diet. There are basically two kinds of foods.

There are foods that build you up.

There are foods that tear you down.

And sadly, most people eat more of the 'tear-you-down' foods than the 'build-you-up' foods.

Fats, sugar, refined foods, packaged cereals... these tend to be 'tear-you-down' foods.

Fruits, vegetables and salads tend to be 'build-you-up' foods.

You have to get a balance between the two. It is astonishingly difficult in our society to avoid foods that tear you down. But by learning to read labels you can reduce them to a minimum.

I sincerely hope you will do as this brief article suggests. It is my earnest wish for you to never have a problem. Follow my advice, and you will live a long and healthy life. Congratulations.

You have been told you have an enlarged prostate

You realise you have a prostate problem.

You are getting up umpteen times a night to empty your bladder. Your urine flow is slow. It takes ages where it used to take minutes. And even worse, you find all too often that after you have been to empty your bladder, some leaks into your underpants. Not nice!

Listen to these statistics... they're scary!

Did you know that more than 350,000 American men may have to undergo painful prostate surgery this year alone? And many of these men will have devastating side effects.

These include incontinence and impotence.

And I am sure proportionately similar figures will apply to Australia and other western countries.

But the sad fact is many of these men could have avoided this surgery. There are other options your doctor has no idea about.

So let's get into reducing the size of your prostate.

First up, get into the zinc. You must take zinc every single night before you go to bed. Ignore the directions where it says something like 'Take one tablet three times a day with meals'.

That is not the way to take zinc. Take one or two capsules each night before bed. That is the correct way. Zinc binds with elements of your food and becomes unavailable.

Your prostate urgently needs zinc.

Take Saw Palmetto. Take twice the indicated dosage.

Saw Palmetto is a wonderful herb that would seem to have been specially designed by Nature to heal the prostate gland.

It is important to understand that an enlarged prostate is seen as being in a pre-cancerous condition. So it is sensible to take steps to not only reduce the size of the prostate but to also take steps to make very sure the condition does not degenerate into a deadly cancer.

Vitamins A and D are essential for the health of your prostate gland. You can get vitamins A and D in one tablet or capsule. Follow the directions on the bottle rigorously.

It is important to make a habit of taking your tablets. If you only take them when you remember, you will have a problem you don't want. Make a habit of taking them at the same times each day.

These are life-saving habits.

OK. Let's keep going.

The next important supplement for you are the essential fatty acids. These are called Omega 3 and Omege 6. Omega 3 is from fish oils and Omega 6 is from Evening Primrose Oil. It is important for you to take these supplements. They are not easily obtained from the normal western diet.

Taking these Omegas has resulted in significant improvement in many experiments. Men with prostate problems are often deficient in both these Omegas.

The three amino acids (glycine, alinine and glutamic acid) have been shown in several studies to relieve many of the symptoms of Hypertrophy of the prostate. You can usually get these three aminos in one capsule or tablet from your local Health Food store.

Panax Ginseng has a long and honourable record in helping prostate problems. It has been shown to reduce prostate weight and is therefore recommended for an enlarged prostate gland.

Bee Pollen has been used in Europe for over 25 years to treat enlarged prostate and prostatitis. There have been several double blind studies with Pollen showing it is very effective. Scientists do not know how it works. But who cares how it works? As long as it works!

Chew pumpkin seeds. Pumpkin seeds, also known as Pepitas, are great to munch on. They taste good. Don't eat the salted variety, get the healthier unsalted variety.

Pumpkin seeds have a good record in stopping the male dribbling after urination. They are great to nibble. If you have a weight problem then they will stop you from eating the fat-depositing stuff. A snack food that is a healthy chomp!

You will remember in an earlier chapter I mentioned Epilobium. This herb is great for an enlarged prostate. It is also called the small flowered willow, but it's botanical name is Epilobium.

Get into this. It was first mentioned in the book *Health From God's Garden* by the Austrian herbalist, Maria Treben.

Do you need them all? You sure do.

You may have to move out of your comfort zone to take these supplements. Especially if you have always only ever been to a medical doctor for help. But push anyway.

As having an enlarged prostate is very stressful, it is a good idea to take lots of the Vitamin B's. Get yourself a good B complex... you will not usually find these in supermarkets. You need to go to a good Health and Nutrition Centre where they stock a good range of vitamins.

The same dietary advice for preventing hypertrophy of the prostate applies if you have the problem.

Avoid coffee. Drink green tea instead (the Chinese have been doing this for thousands of years and prostate problems are unusual in Chinese males). Alcohol should only be drunk in small amounts. Alcohol will shut off your waterworks as quick as a flash if you have an enlarged prostate.

No sir, your prostate doesn't like alcohol even if you do!

It is important to get your cholesterol level down to a healthy number.

Cholesterol metabolites have been demonstrated to accumulate in the prostate gland... and baby, they are carcinogenic. And that is the last thing you want.

So a word about high cholesterol.

It is the LDL type of cholesterol that causes the damage to our body. This is the one we need to get down. We need the good type of cholesterol, the HDLs.

Now here is something you may have noticed with perhaps a friend or relative with high cholesterol. They have been put on a very low cholesterol diet. Really low.

And guess what! Their cholesterol count went UP and not down. Just the opposite of what was intended. Now, why would that happen?

It happens because your diet provides only around 10 to 15% of your total cholesterol.

Your LIVER provides the rest. A full 85% of your cholesterol comes from your liver. So to get cholesterol down I prescribe Methionine.

Methionine is the amino acid I told you about in an earlier chapter. When it comes to getting cholesterol counts down, it is a marvel. I had one patient whose count was 10 and she came down to 4 in less than three months.

So as part of your therapy and general health, get your cholesterol level down to 4 and below.

As I mentioned at the beginning of this book, I am a great believer in strengthening the host, the body, both physically and mentally.

So eat well. Take the vitamins and other supplements. Get your immune system in full gear… and you will avoid surgery and drugs.

You will find your prostate gland will respond well.

Please re-read this book three or four times. Take notes of the points that apply to you.

It is important that you get into it straight away. Don't put it off.

YOU HAVE BEEN DIAGNOSED WITH PROSTATE CANCER

OK, so you have been diagnosed with prostate cancer… the first thing I have to say is you CAN beat it.

Play the tape two to three times a day. Get it firmly into your unconscious mind. And this applies to the other readers who do not have cancer. You need a healthy mind attitude as much as anyone else.

Read the next chapter on positive affirmations. Read them, shout them out loud. Fill your mind with positivity. Change your focus.

Focus all your attention on getting better. Focus on the end result. See yourself healthy and happy. Crinkle up your eyes. Feel the laughter.

You know, it is true that if you pretend something it becomes real. Act happy. laugh, smile, chuckle, chortle, giggle. Walk with your shoulders back, your head in the air... and even if you felt miserable before, once you do these things, your mood will change.

And your cells much prefer you happy because that makes them happy too. It has been scientifically proven that cells perform much better when you are happy. So get happy.

You must attack. Get off the defensive. Get yourself back in the driver's seat!

Take Bovine Cartilage. This is vital to your success.

Get into the Zinc. The Epilobium. Get into the Saw Palmetto both as a herb and Homeopathically.

Get into the Astralagus and the Cat's Claw.

We are not playing games here, this is serious stuff.

Get hold of Lactoferrin.

Find a Homeopath who can make up Sabal, T4. Carcinosinum and Thymus for you. These are powerful allies and can help you beat the cancer.

Boost your immune system dramatically with Red Clover, Pycnogenol or Grape Seed.

Read this book five or six times. Re-read the chapters you found the most inspiring many times.

It is essential that you take notes. Write down all the remedies I have mentioned throughout this book. By writing them down they will get into your mind and consciousness.

Learn how to do Transcendental Meditation. It has been

proven many times over that people who meditate do much better than those who don't. Deepak Chopra used Transcendental Meditation as part of his therapy at his clinic in Boston, USA.

Read the notes on diet again and again.

Even in crisis times it is sometimes difficult to get one's partner to realise how critical diet is to surviving the attack. Get your partner to read parts of this book. Diet IS critical.

I told you six out of ten people die from diet induced disease! And cancer is no exception. The first step in any curative process is changing the diet.

Develop the habit of eating foods that build you up. Cut out sugar and make a commitment. Taking artificial sweeteners shows you have not shaken off the sugar habit. Cut it cold. No more sugar.

No more fat. If you like salt, then the only salt worthy of the name is Celtic salt. The salt for Northern France, or sesame seed salt. These are pure and natural.

That white stuff we comically call salt is a commercial product. It is bleached with chemicals to make it whiter than white. It has chemicals in it to stop it caking. Chemicals to keep it flowing. It is not a natural product. And this includes a lot of salts sold as sea salt.

If you want to look at the result of all your yesterdays, look in the mirror. We are all self-created. We don't like that thought. We prefer to think that what we see is nothing to do with us. When we have high blood presssure, varicose veins, arthritis, irritable bowel, and yes, cancer... we prefer to think it is bad luck, fate, genes... anything but something we may have had a part in.

But whether we like it or not, we are self-created.

And that is good news. Having the power to create ourselves means we also have the power to change ourselves.

You can do something about your condition. Put on a happy face. Focus on health. Get attention off cancer. Don't be a victim.

Get back in the driver's seat. Take charge of your life. Be the boss. You CAN. YES, you can. Believe me. I know because I have been where you are now.

I know what it is like. I know the agony of mind. I know the feelings of despair and hopelessness.

That is why I know you can beat it.

My dearest wish, my most passionate desire, is for you to beat your cancer.

Please, please, read this book many many times. Take the advice I give you. Take the supplements. Who cares if you rattle?

Do everything. Please!

Then write and tell me you are well again. And that will be the greatest satisfaction I could ever get. I will have succeeded in my dearest hope. I will have put your health, your destiny, your future back where it belongs… in your hands.

They say 'Life is Difficult'. And they are right!

15

How to become the irresistible force against which there are no immovable objects!

But what is difficult for one person is not so difficult for another. I know young mothers with only one child who find it difficult to cope. But I also know young mothers with three children who have no difficulty coping.

What is the difference between them?

It is attitude. It is a frame of mind. It is a way of looking at things. It is a habit. A way of dealing with problems as they come up.

There is a popular saying that goes like this: 'If at first you don't succeed, try and try again'.

And that saying will send you broke. It can destroy your spirit. You have done your best. You have kept on keeping on.

And nothing has changed!

Life is still extraordinarily difficult.

One reason is that the saying, 'If at first you don't succeed, try and try again', is incomplete. It only tells part of the story.

It might be better to listen to another version: 'If at first you don't succeed… you are no different from anyone else!'

But much better is this version: 'If at first you don't succeed, TRY ANOTHER WAY!'

And that is the secret of success in any area

of your life.

Why keep doing what isn't working for you?

Insanity is defined as 'doing the same thing and expecting a different result'.

Think about that. It is brilliant.

And we do it all the time.

When we are ill we rush to the doctor. We get the same antibiotics for everything. And guess what? We find the problem often does not go away. I am reminded of people with skin problems who daub on cortisone creams.

The skin clears... temporarily... then the rash comes back worse than ever. And it does this every time.

And here is the strange thing. It doesn't stop us using cortisone cream. We keep repeating the cycle.

Argumentative people keep arguing with everyone they meet. And lament the fact they have no friends.

Nagging spouses keep on nagging even though it doesn't change anything and eventually destroys the relationship. But they still keep on doing it!

People in business do not give service. They and their staff are rude to people who come into their business... And wonder why sales are down!

What I am saying is it is good for us all to question our behaviour patterns to see if they are working for us.

I BET YOU THINK YOU ARE A POSITIVE PERSON!

Everyone I meet tells me they are positive. Even if in the next breath they reveal they have low self-esteem. And if you have low self-esteem, it is impossible to be positive.

Sick people have low self-esteem. Yes, they do. They will deny it. But get inside their heads and listen to the chat going on.

It is NOT positive. It is negative. It is like visiting someone in hospital. The whole time you are there the only topic of conversation is illness. Not only that of the person you are visiting but you will be told about all the problems of all the other patients in the ward.

All negative stuff.

And negative stuff does not help you to get better. Negative thoughts, and as a result negative attitudes, KILL people.

They hypnotise themselves into the grave.

Seriously. They do. Thoughts become reality.

That is why it is so important to keep a close watch on what you are thinking. You need to tap into your internal chat. You need to be aware of what you are constantly telling yourself.

Let me give you an example. One that happens frequently.

OK. It is Monday morning. And it is a grey rainy day. Sleepily the guy gets out of bed. Only because it is Monday and he has to go to work. Given the choice, he would stay in bed.

Well, there is the first negative thought of the day. No leaping out of bed eager to get into the day. No, a sleepy drag-out-of-bed feeling.

'OH, Not Monday already.'

Then our friend pulls back the curtain and stares miserably at the rain pouring down. He watches mesmerised at the rain streaming down the window.

And the reaction?

'Oh, what a lousy rotten day. You might know, lousy Monday and it is pouring down...' Pictures of wet queues at the bus or train station. Or a difficult drive into town.

All negative. What a start to the day.

And you know what happens? Of course you do, our friend has a terrible day. Everything that could go wrong does go wrong. All because of a negative start to the day.

But if you asked our friend about his attitude I bet he would tell you he is a very positive person.

Because he is not aware of his thinking patterns.

So we have to consciously flood our minds with positive thoughts.

THE SECRET OF THE CHAMPIONS

Champions in sport or business set themselves a clear objective. They know exactly where they want to go and they fully understand what they have to do to achieve their objective.

They are totally focused on winning. They have a mental picture of themselves on the winners' podium receiving their gold medal. They do not allow any negative thought to enter their heads.

No, 'What if I don't win' attitude.

That thought is not allowed to take root and fill the mind with destroying weeds. They focus on what they want and then give it all they have. Everything is poured into that goal.

I know young kids who get up at 5 am winter and summer to go to the pool to swim kilometre after kilometre. And then go to school. Do a day's work there and after school go back to the pool for more coaching. More training. More swimming. More efforts to improve style.

Total focus. A total winner's attitude.

This is why top athletes tend to do so well in Life once they give up the sport as a champion. They are so used to focusing on goals, so used to giving it everything they have, they succeed at whatever they focus on.

And we must do the same.

Our focus has to be health. Our focus has to be surging happiness. Our focus has to be on radiating vitality. Our focus has to be on our internal power to heal ourselves. Our focus has to be on extreme wellness.

We cannot afford the luxury of bad thinking.

We cannot indulge ourselves in negative thinking. It is an indulgence we cannot afford.

But this is hard. It is not easy.

It is far easier to slip into the pit of negative thinking.

Negative thinking fits nicely into what has become our comfort zone. We are preoccupied with our problems.

We dwell on the fact that we have a health problem. Or we worry in case we get one… which is a sure way to attract it to ourselves!

Black thinking seems to be a more natural way to go than to think happy, healthy thoughts. It is just like the way people would rather gossip about someone. Rather pull people down than build them up.

Saying powerful, positive things about other people seems to go against our nature. It is easier to condemn people of a different colour. Easier to condemn a different religion. Easier to find fault than to find something fine in another person.

Easier to brood on past hurts than to forgive. We pick and pick at mental hurts making sure they never heal. No wonder we get sick! This has to change.

If you want radiant health. If you want to be young for your years. If you want your mind and body to give you a healthy body… You must love yourself first.

In my clinic I get quite a lot of overweight people looking for help.

And without exception they all have very low self-esteem. In fact, most people have low self-esteem. Almost everyone you meet would love to have more self-confidence.

People with high self-esteem have self-confidence.

Real self-confidence. Not the outward show of the low self-esteem person. The glitter personality. The showtime person who wants everyone to like him or her.

And high self-esteem is essential to wellness.

You have to love yourself extravagantly before you can love anyone else.

It is said in the Bible: 'Love thy neighbour as thyself'.

And we do!

We find it hard to love ourselves so we find it impossible to love our neighbour. Be that neighbour in another country. In another religion. A neighbour who wears different clothes and talks with an accent.

So we have to love ourselves.

We are told when we are young that to love ourselves is selfish. It will make us proud and conceited. It will give us a 'big head'.

Rubbish! Garbage! Trash!

It is just the opposite.

People with high self-esteem have no need to boast. They know their own worth. People with high self-esteem are sympathetic to other people. They do not try to impress other people. Why would they?

And people with high self-esteem are a lot less likely to get sick than those with low self-esteem.

True!

This is because the person with high self-esteem has a mind flooded with positive optimistic thoughts. It reminds me of the delightful elderly lady I met who told me: 'My doctor told me I had cancer. I said to him, "my dear chap, I **don't have time to have cancer**".'

And that was seven years ago and she is still going strong. And she has never had any medical treatment at all. None!

Her self-esteem is so high she cannot conceive the idea of cancer being in her body. What an inspiration!

But most of us are not that tough-minded. For most of us, no matter how we understand we must be positive, we still find ourselves sliding down the greasy slope of bad thoughts.

It is as though we have no control. And that is probably true. We are mentally out of control.

Deepak Chopra pointed out in his book, *Quantum Healing*, that the DNA has to be reached with positive messages of health.

But what messages are we sending our bodies most of the time?

Messages of ill health.

And this applies to you even if at the moment you do not have any visible signs of disease.

But are you radiantly healthy? Do you leap out of bed, can't wait to get into your wonderful day? Probably not.

OK, OK. WE HAVE HEARD ALL ABOUT THE POSITIVE MIND BUT HOW DO WE GET ONE?

It is one thing to listen to someone going on about the benefits of a positive mental attitude. You can agree with it. It is something you know would change your life for the better.

But how do you get one?

How do we stop the insidious negative thoughts creeping and slithering into our minds? How do we stop them taking over, especially if we have something seriously wrong in our lives?

The first step is to send for the tape I have told you about. Use the order form at the back of the book...all you pay is post, packing and handling. The tape itself is FREE.

This is a powerful tape, believe me. I have used it for the six months it took me to beat cancer. And I still use it everyday. Twice a day at least.

I listen to it while I am gardening. I listen to it while I am washing my car. I listen to it any time I am working round the house. This tape gives you a series of positive messages to listen to.

As you listen, repeat the messages. But personalise them. When the speaker says, 'You want health' for example, say in your mind 'I want health'. And do this all the way through.

This focuses your mind on the speaker's words. It also makes the words personal to you.

And while you are doing this there are subliminal messages on the tape getting into your mind. Subliminal means they are below your conscious level of thought. You cannot hear them.

And this is good because you cannot censor them.

This gets past the negative small voice that destroys us. It is this small voice that Shakespeare spoke about when he had Hamlet say something about thought destroying action. What he actually said was 'The native hue of resolution is sicklied o'er with the pale cast of thought'.

What he was saying is that our determination to do something fades the more we think about it. Because we tend to find reasons why our dreams cannot come true.

It is a classic example of our negative ego doing us in!

So the tape gets past the destructive thinking. It homes into our subconscious. It is one way to get right into our cellular thinking!

So use your tape as often as you can.

What I found after listening to the tape for some time was this. When a negative thought popped into my head, a positive thought whispered 'Rubbish'.

When I was in the Merchant Marine some ships had a gyroscopic compass. When the ship started to wander off course, the gyroscope brought it back onto the set course again.

And after listening to the tape and getting the messages into your mind, it too will act like a mental gyroscope and bring your thinking back on course.

And eventually, positive thinking will become a habit.

Here's more help to beat the blues

To be radiantly healthy, to be able to beat whatever Fate hands us, we have to be positive. We have already gone through this.

But we have to be reminded.

The fire of enthusiasm needs fuel.

I do this with little cards I carry with me all the time. Each card has a positive thought written on it. I look at these cards several times through the day. This keep me on the right mental track.

These cards, these thoughts, keep me focused on my objective of total wellness. Brilliant good health. Totally healthy.

I find it a good idea to have a positive thought ready to bomb any negative thought that rears its head in my mind.

Negative thoughts have a slippery way of sliding under our

guard and into our mind. Once there, if not checked, these thoughts attack our positive thoughts.

Let me explain a little more...

Let's say you have a serious disease. Let's say you are taking all these great alternative supplements. Things are going well.

But that doesn't stop a slimy thought from slithering in.

'What if they stop working?' 'Perhaps it's a fluke.' 'What if I become resistant to the supplements?'

So on and so on.

So you need to have a club ready to bash the negative thought as soon as it appears. Wham! Bash! Pow! Out you go.

I do this with my little cards. And I have a good thought ready to whip into my mind at the first sign of a negative one trying it on!

So what I would like to do right now is give you a list of positive thoughts. Take from these whichever you will.

Write one on separate cards and paste them where you can see them.

Let them constantly remind you of your objective.

By the way, these ideas work for any objective. Not only for health. There is more than one way to use these thoughts.

The best is to shout them out loud. Get somewhere on your own where you don't feel embarrassed.

Yell out… and this is very important, yell out with **passion**.

It is important to put *feeling* into it. Emotion charges the thought with energy. And energy is what you need to make the thought part of your very tissues.

If you cannot find a private place where you can let it all hang out, then whisper the thought out loud — as passionately as you can.

But whenever you read these thought THINK passion. Think emotion. Get a feeling inside you of enthusiasm for what you are reading.

This is powerful stuff. This is the way Champions in any sport work. They power themselves with positive messages tied into their goals. It is a habit. That is why they keep on keeping on. It is a habit.

And it is a habit you can easily learn.

And it will change your life.

So, OK here are some thoughts for you... take your pick.

But be sure to write them down. Carry them with you. Look at them often. Say them to yourself. Make it a habit and watch negative thoughts go out of the mental window.

Are you ready? OK. Let's go...

Look at me, HEALTHEE!

Look at me Cancer Free!

Healthee That's ME!

Cancer Free, That's ME

Never, never, NEVER give in

Yes, YES, YES!!!

I CHOOSE health (or wealth or whatever you want from Life)

I CAN DO ANYTHING! YES I CAN!

Health is flowing to me RIGHT NOW!

Every day, in every way, my life gets better and better

I see possibility where others see impossibility

I do whatever it takes to get where I want to be

I have tremendous self-confidence

I love myself more and more every day

I forgive. I forgive. I forgive... myself and others

I have a fantastic healthy body

My body is strong and healthy

I control my thoughts

Nothing has any power over me

I am a WINNER

I can because I KNOW I can
I feel supremely CONFIDENT
I am packed with lots of powerful ENERGY
A tremendous river of success and happiness is flooding my Life
Every cell in my body vibrates with health
Every day sees me nearer to my goals
I feel more and more self-confident every single day
I count my blessings every day...
Abundance is my natural state
I do whatever has to be done... whether I feel like it or not!
I focus on my goals all the time. They are happening now.
Everything is flowing my way
Healing energy fills my mind and body
I am one with the energy of the Cosmic Mind
My heart is full of love
I only do what is best for me
I am pleasantly relaxed
Nothing bothers me
I take life in my stride
I feel incredibly happy
I always feel cheerful and optimistic
My life is worthwhile
I do whatever it takes to get perfect health
My life is an incredible journey
Kindness and love dominate my life
I feel terrific
Each day I get healthier and healthier

I have my own unique place in the Universe
I only do what is worthwhile
I am happy to be alive and well
I radiate self-confidence
I am a creative person
I am strong
I am filled to overflowing with vitality
I am full of courage
I am calm and serene
I am in touch with my innermost self
I am one with the Universe
I have found inner peace
I am calm and relaxed at all times
Nothing bothers me
I am part of the Universal Plan
I want health… I have health

You can make up your own affirmations. Write down what you want most right now.

It could be health. It could be money. It could be love. It could be almost anything.

Write it down.

Now turn it into an affirmation.

Let's say you want to be rich. You are fed up with having too little money. So you take a piece of paper and write down just how much money you want.

It could be $1,000 a week. It could be $500 a week.

Just put down whatever it is you want.

Now, turn that into an affirmation. Always write your affirmations in **present** time.

Do not affirm 'I am **going** to be rich'. This is because the word 'going' indicates the future, not the present. So you will always find wealth eluding you… you want it in the future. So rather affirm 'I AM rich. I receive $1,000 every week for my work'.

You can apply this technique to anything at all. 'I meet only friendly people' for example. 'I love mixing with other people. I find them fascinating.' And so on.

To add real power to your affirmations, VISUALISE them as already happening.

Sit down. Listen to your breathing. In. Out. In. Out.

Silently make your affirmation with emotion and see it in your mind as already happening. If you have a problem visualising just get the feeling of it happening. This will work just as well.

Let's say you are using the affirmation: 'Every cell in my body vibrates with health'.

Say this quietly to yourself with immense feeling.

Picture your 50 trillion cells alive with electricity. See them glowing and sparkling. See them vibrating with glowing health. See your whole body radiating light from your cells. See every part of your body shooting out light. Feel the light flowing through every cell.

Your cells are brimming over with health and light. See them.

Do this with your affirmation. This is really powerful stuff.

Let me leave you with this thought. I know you can win. I know you can achieve anything you want from Life.

I know you can have glowing health.

I know, because I have done it.

And what one person can do, so can another.

As a friend of mine says 'God doesn't play favourites'.

What works for one works for all… as long as they follow the plan.

You have a plan for perfect health in your hands.

Please use it.

Start right now. Today!

Your general health is most important

It is expecting a lot to be a vital, sexually potent male if you are an overweight person who smokes and drinks too much. If you have high blood pressure, your cholesterol level is over the top, you have hardening of the arteries...

It is impossible to radiate good health if you are unhealthy.

Whilst that seems obvious, it amazes me how many men come to me expecting some sort of miracle. How can they continue with a destructive lifestyle and somehow become super studs? The simple answer is you can't!

Come on, be reasonable. You have to take steps to get well. The fact of impotence itself indicates something is wrong. Well, it does, doesn't it?

So cut down on the fat and fried foods. Cut down on alcohol, give up the cigarettes. Life will still go on! Eat more fruits, salads and vegetables. Drink pure water.

Take care of your body. Where will you live when this body of yours packs it in? Look after it. It doesn't ask all that much.

Do some physical exercise. Do special exercises for your sexual prowess... yes, there are some.

One of the most popular was devised by a man called Arnold Kegel. He is famous for the exercise he developed. He developed it for women with pelvic muscle weakness but found it was equally effective for men with sexual problems.

The exercise is simple. All you have to do is contract the muscle between the anus and the perinium. If this sounds complicated, it isn't. All you have to do is contract your backside, the way you do to stop the flow of urine.

Try it next time you empty your bladder. Stop and start the flow by contracting these muscles. You can contract these muscles any time. Sitting, standing, in public or in private. No one can see you do it.

Start off doing it a few times. As these muscles get stronger, repeat the exercise as often as you can. Do this exercise often during your day.

A bonus is once you get these muscles really well toned, you will have orgasms like your wouldn't believe!

Strong lower back muscles and stomach muscles are essential if you want a happy sex life. So do sit ups, crunches, abdominal contractions and so on. You don't have to do a lot. I am not asking you to become an athlete... just to get some muscle tone there.

You can do it, and you will be glad you did it.

This kind of exercise strengthens the muscles used in sex and also improves the blood supply to this vital area.

16

Overcoming impotence... the secrets to male sexual vitality and superpotency

There is one thing you can be certain of. Men don't boast about being impotent. Men boast about being super-potent, even if they are not!

Could you imagine a man going into his local pub and meeting all his male friends. Could you possibly imagine a conversation something like this: 'Hey, guys, guess what! I have some fantastic news. Yeah, you'll never guess but I am IMPOTENT'.

And all the other men crowd round, slapping their friend on the back shouting: 'Hey, man, that's **good news**!' And turning round shouting to all the other blokes in the bar: 'Hey, isn't it great, good old George is IMPOTENT! It doesn't get better than that!'

No, you will never see a scene like that.

When a man believes he is impotent he keeps it a secret.

He nurses it to his bosom like a black worm with teeth like a piranha. It eats away at him. It grinds into his self-respect. It gnaws at his feelings of self-worth. It gets right into his very sense of being a man.

He pretends to the world at large that all is well. He will even boast of his imaginary sexual exploits to his friends. The last thing in the world he wants them to find out is what he thinks is his dreadful secret.

So let's have a sensible down-to-earth look at this male problem.

Is impotence really just a state of mind?

This depends on which specialist you go to see. Some say: 'It is all in your mind'. Others insist it is a 'mechanical' problem. Something wrong with the function of sexual arousal.

First, let me make one thing very plain to you.

All men go through times when they find it difficult to maintain an erection. In my Naturopathic practice, the men who come to see me with this problem get younger and younger.

I can't dance... don't ask me!

Now there is a real problem for a lot of men when they think they have failed. They think that because they couldn't get an erection their whole world has collapsed round their ears.

They don't realise that this is a common problem. Just like women don't have an orgasm every time they have sex think they may have a problem, so do men who don't get an erection. In both cases this lack of response is perfectly normal.

But things happen!

The man has a deep sense of failure. And no one likes to fail. It isn't the best feeling in the world... But now comes a real problem, especially if he can't get an erection a second time.

Because we don't like failing, we try to avoid situations where we think we might fail. Call reluctance is a familiar problem with a lot of salesmen. This is because they become really down with being turned down again and again.

Because they don't sell on every call, because they get

refused more often than they sell, they feel rejected. They feel they have 'failed'. In reality it could be that the number of sales they make more than compensates for the number of rejections...

But that doesn't matter. We do not like failing... So what the salesman does is this. He finds reasons not to make the calls. He gets over busy with paperwork or he spends too long with customers who do buy, or he spends too much time travelling and not facing up to prospects.

So what has that got to do with sex?

Everything!

Because we don't like to fail, and we mistakenly believe we have failed, we try not to get into a situation where we could fail... so we avoid sexual encounters with our partners!

What do we do? Easy! We go to bed first and pretend to be asleep. Or we do the opposite — we let our partner go to bed and go to bed when we are sure she is asleep.

Some guys even resort to having an argument just before bed so they can stalk off in rage... goodbye to sex. The tricks we get up to are incredible.

But the greatest trick is the one we play on ourselves.

And that is we kid ourselves that it is our partner's fault or that we are genuinely too busy, too tired, too angry, too frustrated... anything but admit that we might have a problem.

This leads to another problem...

A problem that can affect a relationship. Because we want to avoid failure and like to avoid a situation where we might fail, we no longer caress or fondle our partner. Worse still, we push our partner away when she tries to kiss or embrace us.

This is like being asked to dance when we can't dance. 'Gerraway from me' shrieks from our body language.

Our partner cannot understand why she is being repulsed. She then worries she is no longer attractive... and so the relationship goes down a road well travelled. A road we really should not be on.

So let me get this thought into your head. Everybody has a time when they cannot get an erection. Everybody has a time when they cannot keep an erection.

Don't believe the stories these so-called studs tell you. In my opinion, the more a fellow boasts about his sexual prowess the less I believe him. He is shouting too much. People who are confident just get on with things. You don't hear them shouting the odds all the time about how good they are.

True confidence is a quiet thing. It is a sense of knowing. It is not empty boasting. It is not about trying to impress people.

Realise that these guys are like little boys making a noise in the dark to scare away ghosts!

Here is a secret you may not be aware of...

While getting an erection is everything to a male it may not be to the female. There is an old saying that goes like this 'Men want sex... but women, what they want is **love**!'

Think about that for a moment.

What women want is the hugging, the kissing, the caressing, the stroking, the words of affection and love. They want to know you LOVE them, not necessarily that you just want sex with them.

Hey and guess what? While you are doing all this hugging, kissing, caressing and stroking, something warm may happen... wowee!!

Are you prepared for love-making?

Come on soldier boy, are you always ready to make love? The male has so many sexual fantasies it is incredible. One is that we guys should be able to do it any time and any place. So we try to do it when we are full of alcohol. This is a time when desire is high but ability is low. If you are full of alcohol the chances of a good sexual experience can go down the drain.

We try to do it after a stressful day at work. We try to do it when our partners don't feel like it. We try to do it because it is Saturday night and 'we always do it on Saturday nights'. We try to do it when we are getting over the flu, we try to do it after a very late night out and we get home exhausted. But we are game, so we give it a go and not surprisingly, we don't do a very good job of it.

And so we think we have failed...

What a load of rubbish! It is asking too much of ourselves.

Have you heard the male definition of foreplay? It is 'Are you awake?'

Extended foreplay is 'Are you awake? Yeah? Then what about it?'

The French believe foreplay should take **all day**! Yep, ALL DAY!

How about that? Tickling, kissing, saying amorous things, touching, making suggestions. Telling his partner how she is driving him insane with desire... making her feel loved, wanted and powerful... Boy, and doesn't this do something great for sex. By the time you actually get around to it you are so wound up you explode into action.

So if you are not going in for kissing, touching and all those nice things because once or twice you didn't get an erection... get into it.

And the great thing is even if after all you have a real problem your partner will love you more than ever.

Don't give up on love because your penis seemed to give up on you!

SO THERE COULD BE A REAL PROBLEM...
WHAT COULD IT BE?

There are a lot of reasons why a man cannot get the erection he wants. One can be low testosterone. Men with low testosterone are low on desire. They are not craving sex all the time... They may feel inadequate because males with high testosterone seem to want it all the time and can do it all the time.

This is comparing oranges to apples.

We are all biologically individual. And that makes us different.

So let me say this — if you have satisfactory sex once a month it may be that once a month is your cycle. Some men have sex once a week, some once a day... But they have no control over this desire.

I remember years ago when I was in the Merchant Marine one of my shipmates was boasting he was better than I was. His reasoning was that he could grow a moustache and I couldn't. My response was that he didn't grow a moustache. He simply didn't shave and the moustache grew. He had nothing to do with it. And as I was very aggressive in those days I told him he had better find another reason to show he was a better man than me... because I was likely to take him out on deck and pound him!

So it is with sexual desire. It differs from man to man. It is not something over which we have a lot of control. You can't pass a law telling yourself to be able to have and enjoy sex every day or whenever.

You can shout at your penis all day but it won't stand up for you.

So recognise that your problem may be imaginary. It could be that your sexual cycle is different from someone else's. Certainly different from the sexual cycles promoted in some of these 'girlie' magazines where it seems all the readers are supposed to be superstuds.

It's hard to get good sex out of a bad relationship...

What I am about to say can be controversial. It can make some people quite angry... but think about it, anyway.

The sad truth is that a lot of men are castrated by their partners.

Oh, I don't mean they take a knife and do a job on their man. It is a lot more subtle than that.

Everyone knows the jokes about wives and their headaches. Most men know the times their wives went to bed early and were, or pretended to be, asleep when their partner came to bed.

A lot of men know the feeling of rejection when they try fondling their wife and she lies there as though she is not aware of what is going on. Then the man either just gives up or get really wild... and we get marital rape. By the way, I am not justifying marital rape. Forcible sex is not what I am about at all.

But hold on to his thought for a moment... Most of the customers who visit prostitutes are married. Seems the single guys can get all they want for free! (That probably is not true, but it is what a lot of married men believe.) Why do these men go to prostitutes? To get 'affection' and sex they cannot get at home. For some men even synthetic love is better than no love at all.

But for a lot of men the options they take with an unresponsive wife are masturbation or grin and bear it. But the resentment goes deep. And sooner or later, the man stops trying. He gives up on his partner.

But he may not give up on sex. Depending on circumstances he may eventually leave to find someone more responsive... and yet another relationship bites the dust.

But here is a strange thing. When the female wants sex she seems to expect the male to react instantly even if she has been rejecting him for weeks on end. And the male will often do his best. But often he feels he is being used. And then problems with erections can arise. His subconscious mind registers a protest by not putting something up.

Whichever way, it is not good for a relationship.

This book is not long enough to go into all this in any detail. But sufficient to say it is not unusual for a man who feels he is impotent with his partner to have no problem at all with a different partner.

I read in one of the Sunday papers how this 70-year-old man was given a potency pill by his doctor... but ran off with someone other than his wife. Now it just may be that the good doctor should have given BOTH the man and his wife a potency pill each.

There is no point in giving either partner incredible potency if the other one has very little... It could easily destroy the relationship and lead to the divorce court.

It may be that before giving one of the partners a potency pill that both partners should be counselled. The female could have a real problem — she is not being bloody-minded about sex. Her vagina may be cold... this creates problems for a man. Why? Because his penis is a heat-seeking missile.

Even if he manages to have sex there is a good chance he will fail simply because there is no heat in the experience. The cold vagina sucks the heat out of the penis and it flops... So obviously, the female has a problem that need looking into. Maybe it is not so obvious.

So a potency pill may be the best thing if only one of the partners has a problem but it could be a disaster if both have the problem... and only one gets a solution!

OK. So let's have a look at other reasons for impotency.

YOU COULD HAVE A PROBLEM AND NOT KNOW IT...

One of the fastest growing diseases in our society is diabetes. And one of the major problems is that a lot of people don't realise they have it.

Diabetes can cause impotence. The accepted medical view is that half of the men with diabetes will become impotent.

So first, let us have a look at the symptoms that could

indicate you need to see a doctor. The most common sign is increased thirst. Suddenly you find you have no trouble drinking glass after glass of water or other liquid. You have an unquenchable thirst.

Another sign is loss of weight. You eat well but lose weight.

Check your diet. Are you a 'sugar buff'? Do you like a lot of sweet things? Do you find you go to bed tired and wake up tired? But when you have your caffeine jab you feel fine... for a while.

If you have any of these symptoms, go to your doctor for tests.

If diabetes runs in your family, get tested.

Untreated diabetes can lead to even worse things than impotence. A major cause of blindness is diabetic retinopathy... And loss of limbs because they had to be amputated is another real risk for diabetics. Grab this one too while you are at it... diabetics have a shorter life expectancy than those who don't have it.

So get to your doctor... and if you have it then have it treated. Do the correct diet thing, work at getting your insulin need down. Manage your problem.

If you do have diabetes and it is affecting your sex life, check your blood sugar levels. When your blood sugar level has a problem so do you. Getting your blood sugar levels right could also get your sex life right.

Of course, having diabetes can cause stress... and we all know what stress can do to people.

Your penis is a blood sucker. It needs lot of fresh hot blood to stay erect. And unfortunately, diabetes can cause problems with what is called 'peripheral' circulation. Peripheral is the outer edges, like hands, feet and penises... If your penis doesn't get enough blood, if your penis cannot keep that blood locked in, you cannot get or keep an erection.

For most diabetics these problems can be solved. You may need to go to a doctor who specialises in these problems. But please, go before the problems is too far gone to solve!

HEY DOC! WHAT'S IN THAT PILL YOU GAVE ME?

Let me tell you a little story about impotence. This lovely man came to see me and told me he had this terrible and shameful problem. He could not get an erection!

'Is it my age?' he asked.

'No, because age shouldn't make any difference to ability, usually only to frequency and time to get aroused?'

'Then what can it be?' he asked.

So as not to bore you... I gave him Homeopathic medicine, I gave him herbs. I tried every darn thing I could think of... but he stubbornly refused to get erections.

Then one day he happened to tell me he had blood pressure problems and was on medication.

'Ahah!' I cried, 'Now we have it!'

Listen to this for a moment. A heck of a lot of blood pressure drugs have impotence as a side effect. One doctor told me he thought that shouldn't be a problem.

'The man is alive isn't he. He should be thankful that he is alive, never mind worrying about impotence... at his age he should be past it anyway.'

Wow, what a great attitude! I bet it would change if he found that some drug he was taking caused his little soldier to faint on parade!

So if you have blood pressure and you are controlling it with a drug, ask your doctor to spill the beans on the side effects. And if one of them is impotence get him to change the drug. If he won't change the drug, then change your doctor!

DOES AGE REALLY MAKE A DIFFERENCE?

A lot of men worry that as they age they will lose their ability to have or even enjoy sex. Women worry that their looks are fading and men worry that their penises are fading.

Has it ever occurred to you that life is just not fair?

Come on guys, statistics don't tell the whole story. Believe the statistics and impotence **triples** between the ages of 40 and 70.

But believe **me** instead. Most of this is the result of a lousy lifestyle.

I tell you what, you would be surprised at the number of men and women who come to see me as patients who are really after something they cannot have.

What is it? They want me to give them something that will enable them to lead a destructive lifestyle and not pay a penalty. And that ain't possible.

The age of miracles has gone. And even if ordinary people could perform miracles with disease they would find themselves in jail for practising medicine without a licence! Wanna bet?

Actually, Life is very fair. We may not think so... But most of the time it is.

We get health problems because we have not done the right thing by ourselves. Poor diet, stressed lifestyle, too much alcohol, poor relationships... all these take their toll of our minds and bodies.

Mother Nature thought of 'play now, pay later' long before the discount houses and the banks.

If you have a destructive lifestyle you may think you are getting away with it for years... but one day you will get the bill. It could be high blood pressure, it could be sludging of the arteries, it could be a million and one medical problems.

But it is never too late to change.

Let me tell you a few things about ageing. Firstly, and this is important, most times when we talk about ageing we are talking about disease.

My ambition is to die young... but I want to be over a

hundred when I do it!

Let's take the average Joe. Here's how it goes... He gets out of bed feeling woeful. Staggers into the bathroom and does what he has to do. He gets dressed, either grabs a cup of coffee and a piece of toast... if he has the time he will sit down to a feast of bacon, eggs, sausages... and even fried bread (maybe only on Sundays!).

Then it is off to work. The journey if he is going by car can be like a Le Mans race. Blast off first at the traffic signals, dodging in and out to get to the front, changing lanes, cursing when the traffic lights are against him, spitting foul oaths at all the idiots who drive cars these days... Hardly a stress-free way to start the day.

His day at work can be stressful too. Even trying not to perform at work can be stressful.

Anyway, good old Joe gets through the day. He finally arrives home frazzled but nothing a couple of beers won't fix. He has something to eat, probably couldn't tell you the next day what he ate, and slumps down in front of the television.

Then to bed old sleepy head...

This is a very destructive lifestyle and leads to an early old age.

It needn't be like that. Take life more easily. Take time to smell the flowers and notice the sunsets... Breathe more deeply. Eat simply of good wholesome foods. Give your body a chance.

And above all EXERCISE.

Stretch those muscles. Get into some form of aerobic exercise. Brisk walking is a good idea. You may see things in your neighbourhood you never noticed before. Do light weights. Keep your bones strong by exercise.

We think of age as being stiff... so loosen up.

You can stay young for a very long time... and your sex life can stay younger too.

Sure, you won't be able to do it as often (maybe you didn't do it all that often anyway). You won't find your little soldier saluting every pretty girl that goes by... but what the heck. It may take a little longer or even a lot longer to get aroused, but you will get aroused!

Sex is a very wholesome exercise for young and old.

And whatever your age, remember this... and tell your partner — men who have plenty of sex seldom get prostate problems.

Sex itself is a great form of exercise... Very healthy — physically, emotionally and in lots of other nice ways.

Get into it folks!

OK. OK. So maybe you can't get into it... so let's go to the next chapter and talk a bit more together.

17 It's all in the mind... or is it?

You heard about the guy who went to the doctor complaining about his poor sexual performance. The doctor listened to his sad tale and then said (with a straight face!)...

'It's all in your mind!'

And his patient said impatiently: 'Listen Doc, I **know** it's in my mind. What I want you to do is to get it down into my pants!'

Well, the truth is a lot of men can't decide whether it is in the mind or it is a physical problem.

So here is a little test for you... won't take long and it doesn't hurt (the ideal test!).

Put some ice on your scrotum. Go on, I'm not kidding you, put some ice on your scrotum! Your testicles should beat a hasty retreat and try to climb back into your body. If they don't do this then you could have neurological damage and you need to see a doctor.

Now boys, it is perfectly natural to wake up in the morning... or through the night with a nice big erection. When I was in the Merchant Marine they used to call it being 'piss proud'. The reason for this was that once the guy emptied his bladder the erection disappeared.

So if you are not getting these erections you could have a physical problem and need to consult your doctor.

The other sign of a physical problem is a cold penis. A penis in good condition is warm to hot... to very hot! If you have a cold penis, suspect circulation problems.

While you are there, run your finger along your penis and feel for any hard nodules. If you find some then there is a good chance you have a degree of calcification. This gets in the way of the blood supply and causes problems.

If you find these nodules, then see your doctor, OK?

A CHECK LIST FOR PHYSICAL CAUSES OF IMPOTENCE

If you were to have a check list for impotence problems it would look like this:

- Do you have diabetes?
- Are you well overweight?
- Are you, or have you been, a heavy smoker?
- Do you drink a lot of alcohol?
- Do you have high blood pressure, and are you on medication?
- Do you have a thyroid problem?
- Have you been exposed to industrial chemicals in industry or on a farm? Have you been exposed to any crop spraying chemicals?
- Do you have kidney problems?
- Do you have hardening of the arteries?
- Do you get pains in your legs when walking even short distances?
- Do you have a cold penis?
- Do you find you do NOT have an erection when you

wake up in the morning or through the night?
- Do you have an enlarged prostate gland?
- Have you ever had surgery on your prostate or bladder?
- Have you had radiation on your prostate or chemotherapy?
- Do you have difficulty passing urine, especially in the morning or when you have had alcohol?
- Are you on female hormone drugs?
- Do you have cardiac or vascular disease of any kind?
- Are you on Beta-Blocker drugs of any kind?
- Are there any small lumps in your penis indicating calcification?
- When you have sex do you have any ejaculation problems... like going too soon or not being able to ejaculate? This could indicate a prostate problem.
- Do you have what they call 'abnormal blood leakage'? This means the blood is not held in your penis and drains away too quickly causing a loss of erection.
- Do you have a highly stressed lifestyle?
- Are you tired and depressed? Are you on anti-depressant drugs?
- Do you have a 'high living' diet — lots of sauce, spicy food, meat and so on? This could cause a build up of cholesterol and impede circulation.

Quite a check list, isn't it?

Don't shirk going through it. Naturally, you don't expect to have all the indicators, but then you don't need them all to have a problem.

The fact is that most causes of impotence are physical. I hurry to say that there are a lot of men who do have a mental problem of some kind that causes them problems with sex.

An over-strict upbringing can create problems. I am Scottish and my father used to make the most ridiculous statements about sex. He told us boys that sex was weakening. I must say, I always find sex just the opposite. I feel great after sex!

According to my dear Dad, touching your own body was a sure sign of physical and mental deterioration. In fact, NOT touching yourself is much more likely to indicate some sort of hang-up.

My Dad, being a true Scot, had a Calvinistic upbringing himself and believed this was the only way to think. Like a lot of other people who think they have a monopoly on moral and other values, he was wrong.

Fortunately, my brother and I thought it was a load of old cobblers, a lot of rubbish and chased girls merrily to the disgust of Dad. So we survived this old fashioned stuff... but a lot of people, men and women, do not survive it. They take it in almost with their mother's milk.

They have great guilt complexes about sex.

It is difficult to have a raging erection when you feel with all your being that this is a sure sign you are on the road to Hell!

So some counselling is needed to correct these beliefs.

It is not a bad idea to check a lot of what are called your 'core' beliefs. These are things like: 'To get rich you have to be a crook', 'Hard exercise is bad for your heart', 'Other people can be successful but not me', 'Money is scarce', 'You have to struggle to get anywhere' and so on... check out your thoughts about sex.

And ask yourself these questions:
'Who told you that?'
'Who told you about sex?'
'Whose opinions are you really expressing about sex?'
'Who told you long ago that sex was dirty?'

It is a good idea to Spring Clean your belief closet every now and again. Chuck out the out-of-date beliefs you inherited from a previous generation.

Believe me, you were created to have sex... and as often as you liked... it is intended to be fun... so don't take it so seriously, enjoy it!

IT IS A FACT THAT VARIETY ADDS SPICE TO LIFE!

Monotony kills everything.

I once told my Mum I liked mince and potatoes. That was a mistake. I got mince and potatoes every time my dear Mum ran out of ideas for something to get me for a meal.

Where I used to look forward to mince and potatoes when I was a kid it got to the stage when I exclaimed to myself in horror: 'Oh NO, not mince and potatoes AGAIN!' So like turned to dislike.

It's the same with your sex life.

Doing it the same way time and time again makes it a duty and not fun. Gotta get out of doing things the same way all the time. Drive a different way to work. Mow the lawn in a different direction. When you wash your car, start at the back if you always wash it from the front end.

And the same with your sex life...

Do things differently... and in different places... not the same old boring bed. Put some spice into your sex life.

This may need for one or both of you to move out of your comfort zone. But let me tell you, nothing changes if you stay in your comfort zone.

I have to confess I am a pretty old-fashioned guy... and a Scotsman to boot but let me tell you how I discovered that everyone didn't do things the way I did. I was under the totally mistaken impression that the rest of the world behaved just as I did... especially in the matters of male/female relations.

One day my dear wife came home laughing like mad. She had been out to a coffee klatch with the girls. One of the girls told the rest of them that she loved having a bath with Milton. Let me explain something... at that time a big selling disinfectant was called Milton. All the girls knew of it because they used it to sterilise the baby's bottle.

So they thought it odd that she would put Milton in her bath water.

And they asked her why she put Milton in the bath.

Apparently, she burst out laughing and explained that Milton was the name of her husband!

All the girls at that time, all married women, thought this was exceedingly daring...

So when my wife told me about it I was amazed. It was something that would never have crossed my mind.

So I persuaded my wife to try it.

However, I have to tell you I only did it once. Why? Because I got to sit on the bath plug with my back to the hot tap, that's why!

But that didn't stop us from experimenting in other ways.

Do whatever it takes to get boredom out of your total relationship, not just the sex bit, and your whole life will improve. There is an excellent chance your impotence was purely temporary.

It's all **WHOSE** fault?

If you want to wreck your sex life altogether, have a blistering blaming session with your partner.

You see it all the time. There is that couple at the party and they are busily firing shots over each other's bows all the time. Sniping away merrily. Gotcha, that time... Yeah... and gotcha back twice as good, see!

They put a heck of a lot of effort into putting each other down.

No wonder the divorce courts do such good business.

If there is a sexual problem in a marriage or a relationship, and there often is, TALK ABOUT IT... to each other.

I am not talking about shouting accusations at each other.

A problem so many people have is they can't discuss anything with their partner. It always degenerates into a blaming session.

A fatal word is ALWAYS.

You are always leaving the place in a mess...

You are always making me look small...

A response is often 'Yeah, well give me an example of when I always do it'.

An exchange going nowhere.

So take 'always' in this context out of circulation. Ban it. Chuck it in the bin.

And while you are there, throw out NEVER too.

'You never take me anywhere.'

'You never appreciate what I do for you.'

'You never clean the mess up after you have done something.'

And on it goes, around and around, getting nowhere but creating a lot of heat and resentment.

Now what we need is light not heat.

If you find it is impossible to sit down and talk with your partner about sexual matters without each of you getting angry and into blame-frame, then go see a counsellor. Get help.

This is not a time for stupid pride. Get help... and you will save your relationship and your sex life.

You could come away saying 'Gee, and all the time I thought I was impotent!'

BY THE WAY... HOW BIG IS BIG?

When I was a kid at High School we always tried to have a peek at the other guys' penises. How big were they? Because everybody knew the bigger the better!

We were pretty terrible kids, I can tell you. We used to chant awful rhymes... one of which I will share with you... but don't go around telling people what a dreadful child I was. Here goes...

'Long and thin, goes right in, doesn't please the ladies... Short and thick does the trick — manufactures babies!'

You could say we were pretty advanced sexually for our ages, in those days, anyway.

But the real truth is that size doesn't matter.

Physically, most of the sensitive nerves in the vagina are at the entrance and in about three inches. Most women say penis size doesn't matter to them. Some women like a penis in all the way, but most don't care one way or the other.

They are most interested in the rest of the male anatomy. Your physical shape, muscle tone, cleanliness and these things. Penis size is very much a male obsession.

It is a shame that so many men go through life full of fear because they think their penises are deformed in some way. Did you realise that when erect, most penises are about the same size regardless of what size they were at the starting gate?

So if penis size has been bugging you, don't worry it ain't the size of what you've got, it is what you do with it!

Don't worry, don't hurry, slow starters make great finishers...

Human beings are a strange lot. Women worry about the size of their breasts. Are they big enough, too big, different sizes and so on.

And all a waste of time.

When did you last put a tape measure to a woman's breast or pulled out a chart with average sizes to see how she measured up. Never!

And the same with us men. We worry about things that don't matter rather than getting on with the job and enjoying ourselves.

We think too much at times. Sex is a feeling, sensuous experience — it is not a cerebral exercise. It is a feeling game in all ways.

So relax, enjoy yourself... you have my permission!

Doctor Kegel knew a thing or two!

A problem that is quite common is weak muscles of the floor of the pelvis. This can cause you to dribble when you think you have finished urinating. A strong set of muscles in this department can help you to a healthy prostate and at the same time help your sex life.

The advantage of this simple exercise is you can do it any time and nobody knows you are doing it.

All you do is contract the muscles you usually use to cut off a stream of urine from your bladder. So here is what you do — contract those muscles as tightly as you can. Hold the tension for a count of three. Then let go.

Repeat this exercise for at least twenty times. Try to build up the number of contractions. Do this at least three times a day. More often if you can manage it.

Don't strain. Take it easy. There are no prizes for the number of contractions or the number of times you do it.

Just remember to do it!

Thank you Doctor Kegel!

I've read all that and it is still in mind...

It isn't always a physical problem, this matter of getting a sustained erection.

Let me tell you one of the greatest obstacles is FEAR.

A guy can't get an erection and he thinks there is something wrong. He tries again and misses out a second time...

Horror, disaster, misery and woe.

Fear takes over. He gets to the stage he is afraid to try in case he fails again... So he stops trying.

His body obliges his mind by making failure impossible. The guy can't fail because he can't try... he can't get an erection at all.

Now it is easy to point out that fear is our enemy and should be ignored... but we can't command our penises to stand to attention. Often we can't command our fears to evaporate either.

So a person who has a mental hang up over sex may be better off getting professional advice.

Because this problem CAN be fixed. The worst thing you can do is to keep it all in. Fear that is not confronted grows... and grows. And this is true in every area of our lives, not just the sexual side.

We all need to calm ourselves. To centre ourselves. To listen to the inner singing of our body. It is in silence that we realise truths.

You don't get much insight rocking and rolling...

Deep breathing is essential. Most of us are shallow breathers. When you are nervous or afraid you breath quickly and shallowly. When you are really calm you breathe slowly and deeply.

To beat fear, practise deep breathing. This is not pushing out your chest like a pouter pigeon. The old army style of pushing out your chest and pulling in your stomach is not what you want.

What you want is to imagine you are drawing your breath into your stomach.

When I played Judo I always practised stomach breathing before a contest. I would kneel and put my hands on my thighs and concentrate on drawing my breath into my stomach.

This calmed my mind and got me ready to fight at my best.

When you are afraid you do not operate efficiently. You make unwise decisions.

So it is with our sex lives. Take time to breathe. Take time to feel sensual. Stroke yourself. Gently hug yourself. Let go of tension...

But if in the end, all this doesn't work for you, then drop your fear and go and see someone who specialises in sexual problems.

You can be helped, believe me. The right practitioner will bring your sex from your mind down where it belongs... in your pants!

18 | Here are the secret herbs and other helpers!

These days you can go to your doctor and get a drug to make you a real stud. This drug is so effective that some men have dropped dead from heart attacks while using it.

Now, the less sensitive among us may say 'Boy, but what a way to go!' But if the price of being virile is dropping dead while having a good time, I would be looking elsewhere for a stimulant.

Nowadays, a lot of doctors are demanding the person who wants the drug sign a form accepting all responsibility for any side effects. The doctor is saying I will give you this drug because you insist, but you and not me take the responsibility for any side effects.

Some guys are so desperate they can't wait to get the pen out of their pocket and sign on the dotted line.

But it might be a good idea to try a herbal alternative first!

First, we meet the herbs!

Herbal folklore is full of secret recipes to enhance sexual function. This problem has been around a long, long time, believe me. And what is more, my friend, you are not alone. It is estimated that over TEN MILLION American males have sexual difficulties.

That is a lot of men!

A herb that is often talked about it Yohimbe. This is one herb that even the establishment admit is a sexual stimulant. Yohimbe is not available everywhere. You can get it over the counter in America, but you can't buy it in Australia.

The reason is Yohimbe, whilst doing a good job on the sexual side, can have side effects for some men. It can raise blood pressure. In fact, it has been used on men with low blood pressure to normalise it. It can also cause panic attacks, nausea, headaches and dizziness.

This is not true of everyone who takes it and it has been used for hundreds of years in folk medicine, so a lot of men have had benefits from it.

One of the problems, in my opinion, is that most Yohimbe is actually a chemical extract from the herb and not the whole herb. It is hard to get it through to manufacturers that all herbs have other qualities than just the 'active principle'. Drug companies search for the active principle, isolate it and produce it as a drug.

But the truth is there is more to a herb than just the active principle. And when this is all that is used, other more subtle factors are ignored. Nature works in total and not in isolation. So it would be interesting to discover if using just the herb would give similar side effects.

You can get Yohimbe in Homeopathic form and I have found this works very well, with no side effects.

As someone with a prostate problem it is interesting to hear that Yohimbe does not work by increasing testosterone.

PENILE MUSCLE POWER...

The penis has muscle. OK, so you want it to have more muscle than it appears to have right now... The muscle in the penis is what is called smooth muscle. And it needs to be relaxed not tensed up like a bodybuilder's biceps.

And guess what, there is an amino acid that does just that. This amino acid is called Arginine. I have had wives come in and thank me for helping their men do their stuff. I have found that Homeopathic Yohimbe, in Australia, combined with Arginine, can do wonders. As one woman said 'It hasn't made him into a stud... but things are much better!'

HERE IS ANOTHER HERB TO THE RESCUE...

Have you heard of a herb called Gingko Biloba?

This is one of the most prescribed herbs in Germany where doctors routinely prescribe herbs. They usually give it to students to help improve memory and thus studying...

But it has a lot of other qualities too...

Most people have heard about Gingko for ringing in the ears. They have heard about it for circulation, remedying cold hands and feet.

But not many people realise it is excellent for lovemaking!

You know what, around five million prescriptions a year are given in Germany by doctors over there... but I bet you almost anything your doctor has never heard of it.

And this is really quite surprising when you find how useful it is for helping elderly people who have terrible memory problems. It can help one of our most feared health problems, Senile Dementia or total loss of memory.

But let's get back to sex...

Your penis is a blood sucker, as I have remarked before... and Gingko supplies blood. If you have a problem because there is not enough blood getting to where you want it... then Gingko Biloba could be just what you have been looking for.

I have heard of men who do not have an erection problem but who take Gingko before sex to give them an extra lift.

The beauty of Gingko is that while it improves blood flow through the arteries and veins, it does not affect blood pressure.

Hey, it might just be what your doctor **didn't** order!

How about a herbal alternative to Viagra?

Viagra is big news at the moment. Men are rushing to their doctor and saying anything to get their hands on this latest 'wonder drug'. And there is no doubt it has put new wine in old bottles, taught old dogs new tricks and generally vitalised a lot of lives.

It has also wrecked a few too.

There are stories of marriages failing because the female couldn't keep up with the incredible sexual appetite and ability of her old mate. He has gone off seeking new pastures where he can make hay while the Viagra sun still shines.

But there are reports of men dropping dead while looking for a new lease on life. Because of this very real danger, doctors are demanding that men who want Viagra sign a declaration absolving their doctor from any liablity should the patient do a number on himself.

Great news though... there is a herbal alternative you may not have heard of...

It is called Tribulus.

The reputation gained by Tribulus by those in the know is remarkable. Just listen to this lot, your energy will rise, you will have more stamina, your libido increases (hey, where can I get this stuff?). But there is more! It is a liver cleanser and is said to help menopausal women with their problems.

Quite a remarkable lot of claims.

The full name of this herb is Tribulus Terrastris, commonly called Calltrop Fruit and I am told it has been used for centuries in Europe for hormonal insufficiency in men and women. Just goes to show, it is remarkable what we don't know!

This herb is now out of the closet and into the open. Even the scientists have been having a look at it... And this is what they have found... Tribulus significantly increases the levels of testosterone (so no good to prostate sufferers!) and Luteneizing Hormone. This hormone is a gonad stimulating hormone produced by the Master Gland, the pituitary. It also stimulates follicle producing hormone in women.

It increases sperm production and testosterone levels in men... Seems to me a likely starter for people having difficulty starting a family.

The good news is that no bad side effects have been found using Tribulus. In fact, Tribulus actually improves liver function and could be useful to reduce cholesterol levels. There have been no adverse effects noted on the vascular system... so not much chance of a heart attack when giving it all you've got.

The reported result of taking Tribulus are something men with erection problems have dreamed about... Just give this your attention, increased testosterone after only five days. Increased libido, you feel like it a lot more often. Increased strength of erection... you can keep it up for increased joy.

But it's not all for the boys. Here are some benefits for the female of the species. Increased estrogen and she too will experience greater libido.

On this point, may I say I find it quite disturbing in my clinical practice how many **young** men and women come to me for help with the problem of a low or non libido. These are people who one would expect to be at it all the time... like we were at their age!

Continuing on for the benefit of females... they also have improved ovulation with Tribulus. It reduces hot flashes in menopausal women and also reduces apathy and irritability.

Gosh, some blokes will want to get it in truck loads!

And the beauty of it is you don't need a prescription, you can get it over-the-counter at your health food store.

THE ANCIENT CHINESE KNEW A THING OR TWO...

The Chinese have used Panax Ginseng for thousands of years for male sexual dysfunction. (Don't you just love this modern expression, 'dysfunction' — sounds better than inability.)

Ginseng helps your body to adapt to stresses and strains that make life difficult. So have a look at Ginseng as part of your regime.

Vitamin B3 in the form of Niacin can help. Niacin is a vasodilator — it causes the blood vessels to expand slightly. This enables the blood to flow more quickly. In fact, one of the problems in taking Niacin is that you can get an unpleasant tingling and feeling of heat in your face and body. This passes off after a little while. Best to take it with food to reduce this effect.

YOU MIGHT GO HARDER IF YOU RELAX...

In our modern rush and bustle life one problem we may not realise we have is this... we do not make time for sex.

There is no plan in our lives for love-making. All too often we are dead beat and sex is the last thing we are interested in. This is bad news if your partner is full of life at that moment!

So as I said before, slow down, we'll all get there soon enough.

To this end though, it could be wise to think about taking some anti-stress vitamins. The B group of vitamins are in short supply when we stress ourselves out. So taking a good B could be something to add to your list.

Anxiety is a problem when men find they have erection difficulties. So it may be a good idea to take St. John's Wort, otherwise known as Hypericum. Here is something you may find surprising... in Germany again, doctors over there prescribe as much Hypericum as they do Prozac for anxiety.

So if anxiety is causing you to fail, then taking Hypericum could be very handy indeed.

DRINK FILTERED WATER... TAP WATER IS NOT YOUR FRIEND!

Someone remarked that we live in a 'sea of estrogen'. Here is something that will make you think. Do you know what is one of the major health problems facing our survival on this planet?

First up, we automatically think of super viruses, or Greenhouse gases, or El Nino. But it is none of those things, threatening though they may be.

It is feminisation of the male.

More and more little boys are being born with deformed penises... and not only human boys but the male offsprings of fish and even crocodiles.

Researchers placed a cage full of male fish by the water outflow and after a few months all those fish started showing female characteristics.

This is due to the estrogen in our food supply.

Commercially, giving cattle estrogen in their feed makes good sense. You can get the cattle up to weight faster on less food... which makes more profit.

But you get some of that estrogen when you eat your delicious steak!

Just as you get antibiotics when you eat a lot of factory farmed chickens.

But here is something you probably had no idea about. Some pesticides and other chemicals that get into our water supply act like estrogen once in our bodies.

Now if that doesn't put fear into your heart, nothing will.

Can you imagine the long term consequences of this if nothing is done? We will no longer be able to reproduce as a species...

Armageddon will arrive and we will not realise it!

My own defensive tactics are simple.

I am a vegetarian and I only drink filtered water.

It may be a good idea for you to do the same...

You've tried all the herbs and still no luck!

It could be you have some kind of structural damage to your most vital organ, so what can you do now?

Don't give up hope just yet.

If you are game there are other options, the major one being implants of different kinds.

These come in a few different forms... The general way this is done is by a medical practitioner inserting a rod into the penis. Some are permanently stiff, so the man has a sort of semi-permanent erection. Others come erect when you squeeze a little bulb hidden in the scrotum.

It is best to look for professional advice if you think an implant is the answer.

A FEW LAST WORDS ON SEX AND SEXUAL ABILITY... AND IMPOTENCE

Remember this — when a man ages it takes longer to get aroused. Young men have no problem. Their little soldier leaps to attention at the slightest provocation and is action-ready in seconds.

But as we age it takes longer. Our battle-weary soldiers need a little more persuading to come to attention. But with patience, a lot of love play (and what's wrong with that?), he will finally get the idea and stand up to be counted.

Of course, when we are younger we cannot imagine a day coming when we would have difficulty saluting every girl who goes by. But as Bette Davis was quoted as saying 'Growing old takes guts'... But more than that, it takes knowledge, and that is what you have got here!

Basic things are eating proper food. A good diet can make for a good sex life. Don't clog up your system with junk. Drink plenty of clean water. Eat plenty of fresh vegetables, fruit and salads.

If you have a lot of gas, get your digestion checked out. You can't function in any department if your system is fouled up.

A FEW FINAL WORDS...

I wrote this book with only one thought in mind.

To help my fellow men avoid the disaster that happened to me. To give hope and courage to those who are experiencing the despair of prostate problems.

It is of great concern to me that when a man presents with a prostate problem, the options offered are so restricted... and in many ways, very unpleasant. It is my mission to bring to all men the facts so they and their loved ones can make an informed decision about their medical future.

I believe that after reading 'How To Fight Prostate Cancer and Win' you will be in a vastly improved position to do something positive about any prostate problem no matter how bad or frightening it may be.

If I have made you think, if I have inspired you with hope and courage, if I have given you information that has been a revelation to you... and if you follow my plan and do as I did... WIN... then I have done what I set out to do.

We are comrades, you and I, strangers when we met at the beginning of this book, friends at the end of it.

Thank you for investing in my book.

You can help me spread the word to the ever-increasing number of men suffering with prostate problems of different kinds by telling them about my book and where they can get it.

I would thank you for this... but not as much as the man to whom you introduce my book!

HERE IS A LIST OF NUTRIENTS I TALK ABOUT

Please note: The nutrients which are very helpful for almost any illness or disease (especially serious diseases) are marked with asterisks.

*Acidopholus	Taking youghurt is not enough. You need to totally repopulate your bowel. I use Flora boost by Health Wise because each capsule contains 10 billion friendly bacteria. I take one capsule three times daily before meals.
*Antioxidants	I took the pine bark/grape seed combinations with vitamins A, C and E.
***Astralagus**	A lot of health professionals claim that Astralagus is good for any kind of cancer. I take 1,000 mg at least three times a day.
*Betacarotene	I use the 25 mg strength and take at least 2 a day.
***Bovine Cartilage**	This with Lactoferrin are the two most powerful of anti-cancer nutrients. *Refresh your memory by going back to page 157 to read about this powerful anti-cancer nutrient.*
	The bovine Cartilage I use and recommend is called *OxyMin Flex*. This is strong and excellent quality. Take one teaspoon a day as a preventative. If you have a health problem take at least one teaspoon three times a day.

*Cats Claw	This South American herb is great for any serious illness and as an immune booster. I take two capsules three times a day.
*Co Enzyme Q 10	This is the 'spark plug' of the cells. It is wonderful for energy and you need energy to fight any illness or disease. Take as directed on container.
*Colon	It is very important for good health to keep your colon working properly. Flaxseed, Linseed, Psyllium Husks, Slippery Elm Bark powder, Oatbran are all good. Unprocessed bran is too rough for some people.
	I recommend a product manufactured here in Australia called "Quick Fibre Plus". This product contains all of the above natural ingredients, which have been ground and blended carefully together in precise proportions. You simply mix 1 or 2 tablespoons in 200mls of soymilk every morning for breakfast
Epilobium	This is also especially good for the prostate gland.
*Flaxseed Oil	You get Omega 3, 6 and 9 from flaxseed. This is important for any disease, but especially so for sufferers with prostate problems. I take the capsule form, one capsule three times a day
*Ginseng	This is a great tonic for prostate or any other condition where more vitality is needed. Get

Panax, not Siberian. Take as directed on container. Do not take with Vitamin C.

***Homeopathy** You will have to find a good Homeopath for these medicines. Whilst Homeopathy has been used very successfully for over 200 years it is still sneered at by the Medical Profession. The remedies you need are Carcinosinum, Cancer (if you have cancer), Thymus and T4. A good Homeopath will also make up for you your Constitutional remedy which will help any health problem.

*Lactoferrin This is a most remarkable substance and something I recommend to all my patients and readers. *Refer to page 174 to refresh your memory.*

The Lactoferrin I use is *Health Wise Lactoferrin.* For prevention take one capsule once a day. If you have a health problem then take at least three to six capsules three times a day.

Lycopene Lycopene is found in tomatoes, but they must be cooked. You can either eat lots of tomato paste with your pasta or take capsules. Follow directions on container. The capsules I rake are Healthwise Menz, This formula has 5 mg of standardised natural Lycopene. This is a therapeutic dos. Most other formulas have only 2 mg of synthetic Lyocpene which is not of any real value to you..

*Methionine	This amino acid is excellent for the liver, for reducing cholesterol and general health. I take the powder form, half teaspoon in water, at night and in the morning.
*Pau d'Arco	This South American herb has a great reputation for helping with cancer of any kind. Take as directed on container.
Red Clover	Taken for its Geniston content. You can get this as Red Clover or under a brand name. Valuable for prostate gland and cancer.
Saw Palmetto	Also called Serenoa or Sabal Serrulata. This is critical for the prostate gland. I take HealthWise Menz which has a therapeutic amount of Saw Palmetto in each capsule.
*Selenium	This is one of the most important anti-cancer trace elements. It is freely available in the U.S.A. but not in Australia. In Australia you can either get a doctor to prescribe it or get the Selenium ACE powder and take a teaspoon two or three times a day in water. Do not think that more is better. Selenium is toxic in large amounts!
*Vitamin C	I use the powder form so I can get a lot at one time. Mix it with water (pure). I take at least 5 grammes a day... when I was ill I took 20 grammes a day in divided doses.
*Vitamin E	I take 1,000 i.u. a day. This is 2 capsules.

Zinc — Zinc is essential for a healthy prostate gland and male reproductive system. The instructions on most containers of zinc are incorrect. You should not take zinc with food. It is best on an empty stomach/to take either last thing at night or first thing in the morning.

A WORD ABOUT THE AMINO ACIDS ALANINE, GLYCINE AND GLUTAMINE.

One of the signs of a prostate problem is getting up umpteen times through the night to empty your bladder. It is also a sense of great urgency when you need to use the toilet, so much that quite often the poor man has the embarrassing experience of wetting himself. The other embarrassing experience when you have an enlarged prostate is standing there in the urinal like forever waiting for the flow to start.

Research revealed that the three amino acids Alanine, Glycine and Glutamine have remarkable success with these bladder problems. They reduced the night-time urination in 95% of the men in the study. Urgency was reduced in 83%, frequency reduced in 73% and having to stand and wait for the flow to start, reduced in 70% of the men.

IMPOTENCE HELP

Arginine — This amino acid is available from your local Health Food Store. Take as directed on container (take it with your Yohimbe).

Ginkgo Biloba — This is a great herb for circulation problems. Take as directed on the container.

Ginseng   Use Panax, take as directed on container.

Tribulus   This herb is going to be one of the most popular around. Ask your Health Store for a brand that has both root and fruit in it as this is the most potent. Take as directed on container.

Yohimbe   This is freely available in the U.S.A. but not in Australia. However, you can get the Homeopathic kind at your local Health Food Store. Take as directed on container.

If you have a problem obtaining any of them, contact Natural Health Direct on 1800 770 771 or email: mail@naturalhealthdirect.com.au.

Once again, thank you for investing in 'How To Fight Prostate Cancer And Win'. Please tell a friend about this book... you could be doing them an enormous favour!

If you need more information or have any questions please see my website at; www.rongellatley.com

Here is a list of nutrients I talk about

Do You Have These Signs Of An Unhappy Bowel?

You will be astonished to discover that a lot of diseases, which seem to have little to do with your bowel, are actually caused by a bowel suffocating with undischarged wastes.

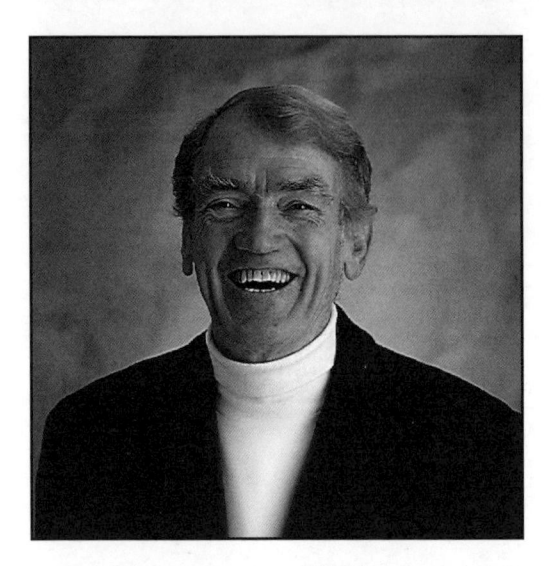

"To See How Well Your Bowel Is Working Check This List".

- Are you constipated? A major cause of ill health.
- Do you have Irritable Bowel? Causes of a lot of misery.
- Do you have Diverticulitis? This is painful, ask anyone who has it!
- Are you embarrassed by wind and bloating? Wind can be a real social problem too!
- How well does your liver work? Irritability, tearful, low motivation, mild depression..these can be liver symptoms.
- Do you have heartburn and other signs of indigestion?
- Are you overweight? Surely a very real problem for lots of people.
- Do you have mysterious aches and pains? You can have aches and pains you do not realise are caused by an unhappy bowel.
- How alive-looking is your skin? Has it a good colour or does it lack lustre?
- How is your cholesterol level?
- Do you suffer from low energy and low vitality?
- Are you crippled by migraines, sick headaches?
- Do you suffer from Thrush (Candida)?
- Do you have backache? You can have one or many of these signs of an unhappy bowel.

If you are like most people, you take these symptoms of an unhappy bowel for granted. You think these problems have other causes. You do not realise that the trouble is really a clogged up bowel choking on wastes that should be in your toilet and not your body tissues.

Imagine how much better your Life would be if you had the secrets of a healthy, vital bowel unclogged with putrid wastes!

The Staggering Truth About Your Bowel And How It Affects You!

What I am about to say may seem way over the top. But it isn't. It is a fact. Did you realise that most diseases gain entrance to your body through your bowel? A healthy bowel is your first line of defence against disease-causing bacteria. A sick bowel actually breeds the bacteria that harm you!

It is a truism to state that Death begins in the bowel. By the way, old age also can start with an unhappy bowel.

Are you beginning to see why it is so important for you to take steps to a healthy bowel? Not only your bowel, but also your liver, your digestion, getting rid of parasites.

How can you be full of joy if your bowel is full of wastes which are slowly poisoning you! Think about it! How can you be happy if you have Irritable Bowel, if you are constipated, if you are embarrassed by wind, if you have constant indigestion?

The answer is you can't!

Let Me Show You The Easy Way To Vibrant Health and Happiness

My new book "Internal Health". The Key To Eternal Youth and Vitality (already a best seller) cuts through all the hype like magic. I explain in a simple, down-to-earth way, how to prevent these problems from spoiling your life. And even more important, I reveal to you little-known ways to beat these problems if you are suffering from any of them.

As one reader said "I saw myself on every page. I learned more from "Internal Health" than from 23 similar books I have read".

Here are some of the things you will discover..

- You will find natural ways to rid yourself of constipation for ever.without harsh laxatives!
- You will find simple ways to beat Irritable Bowel Syndrome.
- You will discover "the vitamin" essential if you suffer from Diverticulitis.
- Find out why you don't have to put up with bloating, wind and indigestion if you don't want to.
- You will be surprised to find out why some fibres can make constipation worse instead of better.
- Find out what antibiotics can be doing to you.
- Discover why children who have a lot of antibiotics always seem to catch everything going about.
- Find out what to do if you have been on antibiotics. This is very important information.
- Why eating yoghurt will not do for you what you think it is doing. This is just a fraction of what you will find out in this remarkable new book. Would you like to stay younger longer? Would you like your life to be overflowing with health and lasting vitality?

"Internal Health" is a book that everyone who is serious about their health should have. We have received hundreds of letters from grateful readers who have seen their problems disappear, often after years of trying other ways without success.

Look at some of the comments about "Internal Health" from other people who have read it.

"Recently I purchased your latest book ("Internal Health") and found it an enthralling publication, especially your great humorous way of keeping one interested in the various chapters" and this excerpt.

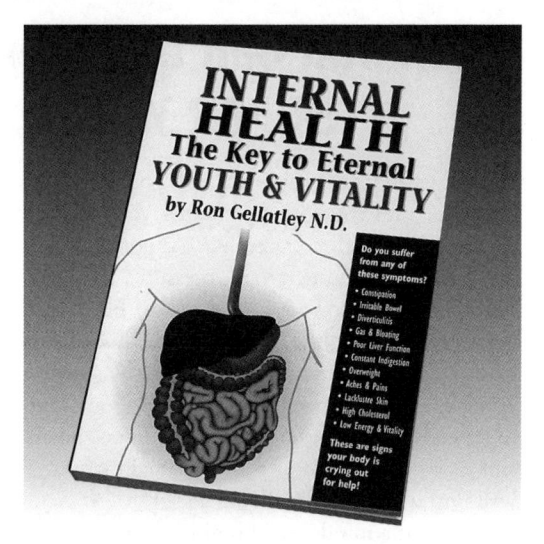

"I have just finished your wonderful book and am, of course, very enthusiastic to preach to the masses".

I have had hundreds of letters praising "Internal Health" from people who have found answers they have been looking for years. As the writers do not want the world to know their problems, I have to leave the quotations from their letters without identification. But we have files bulging with letters all praising this incredible book.

If you suffer from diverticulitis, constipation, Irritable Bowel, bloating and wind, let me show you step-by-step how to free yourself from these problems naturally, without drugs.

The secrets to radiant health, youthfulness, joy and wellbeing are here for you.

I urge you with all my heart to send for "Internal Health" TODAY, do not delay. Why suffer if you donít have to? It makes good sense for you to fill in the coupon NOW or order by phone, fax or Email.

www.cargelpress.com.au
Copyright 2000 Quick Results Marketing Australia

Cargel Press International, Unit 3, 2 Frank St Wetherill Park NSW 2164. Please complete the Coupon and mail to: PO Box 484 Helensvale QLD 4212 or Ph: 1800 632 305, Fax: (02) 9756 0719. Allow 14 days for delivery. Yes! Please Rush me 1 copy of ""Internal Health"...The Key To Eternal YOUTH & VITALITY" @ $32.95 plus $8 Postage & Handling (Total $40.95). Make cheques payable to *Cargel Press.* PLEASE PRINT YOUR DETAILS.

Please charge my ☐ Mastercard ☐ Bankcard ☐ Visa ☐ American Express
Card No. ☐☐☐☐ ☐☐☐☐ ☐☐☐☐ ☐☐☐☐   Expiry date:................ Cheque/Money Order: $............
Name:... Signature:..
Address:.. Suburb:.......................... State:........... P/C:............
Phone: ( ).. Fax: ( )..
2101INT.HE.TELIS.10.00

"Now You Can Discover The Hidden Secrets of SUPER YOUTH....At Any Age!"

As you get older you want to look younger than your age, a lot younger! You want lovely smooth skin, not wrinkled or crazed like old pottery. You want to have young blood pressure, a sound heart, good lungs. You don't want to be out of breath tying your shoe laces like some poor folk!

You want to be free of problems such as diverticulitis, irritable bowel, constipation. You want to rejoice in free movement of your joints, able to still play golf, tennis or run up a flight of stairs well into what people call 'old age'.

You want a mind free of brain fog or fag. You do not want the mists of Alzheimer's Disease to cloud your memory. You want to remember where you leave your glasses or car keys. You do not want to find you cannot remember important things like birthdays, anniversaries......shopping lists.

You want a mind receptive to new ideas, not a mind creaking and stiff. You want to be able to cope with change...indeed, welcome it! You want a flexible mind.

In short, you want to be fit and healthy until the day your die!

"What Most People Call 'Old Age' Is Usually Disease!"

What picture do the words 'old age' conjure up in your mind?

I bet it is one of a white-haired old person, stooped by age, stiff and wrinkled. On lots of medication too without a doubt. High blood pressure tablets, heart tablets, tablets for the pain of arthritis.....an all too familiar story...Tablets to counteract the tablets....not a pretty picture, is it?

"This Is Not Necessary..And Needn't Be The Story Of YOUR Life!"

One of the secrets of living a long life is to harness the power of your mind. In fact, a most important one.. What you think dominates your life to a degree most people are not aware of. 'As you think so you are' is an eternal truth.

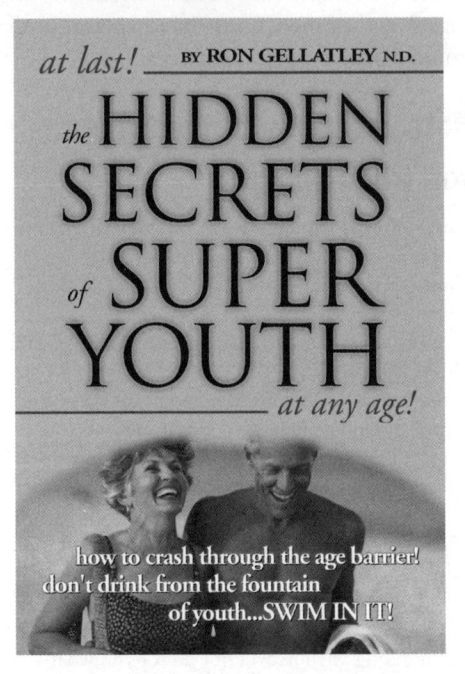

People who live a long healthy life expect to. Most people don't! They actually expect to suffer the pangs of age as the years go by.

Taking steps NOW to make sure your body is kept in peak condition is essential to a happy and healthy old age. When should you start doing things to makes sure you are still vital and active no matter what age you are? The answer is NOW! Not tomorrow or next week, but right now!.

"Amazing New Book Tells You Step-By-Step How To Be Happy, Healthy And Successful........ At Any Age!"

Happiness is essential if you are to be healthy as you age. It is difficult to be happy if poverty stalks you. It is difficult to be happy if your mind is bogged down in the swamp of negative thinking. And the tragedy of negative thinking is all too often we don't even know we are thinking negatively. But we reap what we have sown whether we realise it or not.

In my new book **"At Last! The Hidden Secrets Of Super Youth At Any Age"**

I show you how to program your mind for success, health and happiness. I discuss with you the secrets of all successful people. How they gained wealth, happiness and success. I show you how to stop being manipulated by other people. I show you how to get things done when they should be done. I reveal to you little-known, easy-to-do secrets that can transform your life....no matter how old or how young you are right now.

I show you how to prevent the diseases that plague our modern world. Bowel problems like Irritable Bowel, Diverticulitis, Constipation. How to prevent Alzheimer's Disease and keep your mind young and flexible all your life. I show you how to prevent getting the world's fastest growing disease, Diabetes.

I show you ways to prevent getting arthritis. How to avoid high blood pressure, high cholesterol and all those other complaints we think are inevitable...

"I Not Only Show You How To Prevent These Health Problems, I Also Reveal To You Little-Known-Ways To Beat Them"

My new book is actually THREE books in one.

The first book is about motivation. How to easily train you mind to work for you instead of against you. How to ATTRACT wealth and prosperity into your life. I reveal the thought habits that make it possible for anyone at any age to be rich and successful.

Yes, there are definite thought patterns you can use to transform your life.

I show you how to welcome good fortune, brilliant health and happiness into your life.

The second book is all about prevention. All the secrets you can use to make sure you do not develop the ills and aches of our modern lifestyle. A life free of pain and suffering. I take each of the modern diseases, yes even cancer, and show you how you can keep them out of your life.

The third book is all about what to do if you have health problems you want fixing. Tired of drugs? Tired of being sick? Fed up with getting slowly worse instead of better?

Find out what to do about cancer, bowel problems, diabetes, arthritis, memory loss.....even over-weight....It is all here waiting for you in **"At Last! The Hidden Secrets Of Super Youth......At Any Age"**

This book is an investment in Life itself....YOUR LIFE.

Don't waste a minute, let me give you the advice I would give you if you were my own flesh and blood....get your copy TODAY......I know you will be so glad you did.

Warmest wishes to you, my friend

Ron Gellatley ND

Cargel Press International, Unit 3, 2 Frank St Wetherill Park NSW 2164. Please complete the Coupon and mail to: PO Box 484 Helensvale QLD 4212 or Ph: 1800 632 305, Fax: (02) 9756 0719. Allow 14 days for delivery. Yes! Please Rush me 1 copy of ""At last! The Hidden Secrets of Super Youth, at Any Age" @ $32.95 plus $8 Postage & Handling (Total $40.95). Make cheques payable to *Cargel Press*. PLEASE PRINT YOUR DETAILS.

Please charge my ☐ Mastercard ☐ Bankcard ☐ Visa ☐ American Express
Card No. ☐☐☐☐ ☐☐☐☐ ☐☐☐☐ ☐☐☐☐   Expiry date:................ Cheque/Money Order: $............
Name:.. Signature:...
Address:.. Suburb:........................... State:......... P/C:............
Phone: (   ).. Fax: (   )..
2101INT.HE.TELIS.10.00

"Positive Messages for Vibrant Healing!"

This tape is a powerful tool for vibrant health. All you hear are waves beating on peaceful sandy shores...

But underneath those waves are carefully scripted messages that explode in the force-field of your unconscious mind overpowering negative thoughts and flooding your mind with positive thoughts of health and prosperity...

"You Can Also Have That Tape In Your Hands!"

The tape that has done so much for me is now available to you for FREE! All you need to do is complete the coupon below and post it to Cargel Press with $8.00 to cover Postage and Handling.

I am extremely happy to be able to provide you with this tape. Because my dearest wish right now is for you to get well. I pray with all my being for you to get well.

Cargel Press International, Unit 3, 2 Frank St Wetherill Park NSW 2164. Please complete the Coupon and mail to: PO Box 484 Helensvale QLD 4212 or Ph: 1300 555 337, Fax: (02) 9756 0719. Allow 14 days for delivery. Yes! Please Rush me 1 FREE cassette tape of "Positive Messages for Vibrant Healing". Please include $8 for Postage & Handling. Make cheques payable to: *Cargel Press*. PLEASE PRINT YOUR DETAILS.

Please charge my ☐ Mastercard ☐ Bankcard ☐ Visa ☐ American Express

Card No.

Expiry date:.................... Cheque/Money Order: $....................

First Name:.................................. Surname:..................................

Signature:..

Address:..

Suburb:.. State:.............. P/C:..............

Phone: (   ).. Email:..................................

3RDED.PROS